The Practice of Electrocardiography

The Practice
of Electrocardiography

A Problem-Solving Guide to Confident Interpretation

Thomas M. Blake, MD

*PROFESSOR OF MEDICINE EMERITUS,
UNIVERSITY OF MISSISSIPPI SCHOOL OF MEDICINE,
JACKSON, MISSISSIPPI*

FIFTH EDITION

Humana Press **Totowa, New Jersey**

Printed in the United States of America. 10 9 8 7 6 5 4 3 2 1

Library of Congress Cataloging-in-Publication Data

Blake, Thomas M. (Thomas Mathews), 1920–
    The practice of electrocardiography / Thomas M. Blake. — 5th ed.
      p. cm.
    Includes bibliographical references and index.
    ISBN 0-89603-261-2 (paperback) 0-89603-292-2 (hardcover)
    1. Electrocardiography. I. Title.
    [DNLM: 1. Electrocardiography. WG 140 B636p 1994]
  RC683.5.E5B56 1994
  616.1'207547—dc20
  DNLM/DLC
  for Library of Congress   93-39587
                                        CIP

Preface

Electrocardiography is a mature discipline, so familiar to both doctors and patients that it's hardly noticed, one of those tests that have always been there, like the white count and hemoglobin, not something one has to think about much, or question. To some extent this view is valid, but it overlooks some important points. Like the white count and hemoglobin, electrocardiograms are produced by technicians using mechanical devices that turn out numbers, but there is a difference. The white count and hemoglobin are reported as single values to be interpreted by the doctor who knows the patient and ordered the test, but the graph produced by an EKG machine represents millions of numbers displayed as *XY* plots, a message written in a language different from one's own. It requires translation, and this means that the translator must not only know the language, but also be able to assess the effects on it of the many factors that may have modified its meaning between origin and delivery. There is potential for harm to the patient, as well as for help, in every facet of the process, and to lose sight of this, to see the tracing as a single whole, would be like seeing words as units without considering the letters that compose them. When we read, we do recognize whole words, patterns, but, having learned the letters first, revert to this base intuitively when we encounter a new word, or one that is misspelled.

Electrocardiography is probably the only medical specialty in which no consensus has evolved on just what data must be obtained, how they should be obtained, or, once in hand, how they should be rearranged into a useful statement of what they mean. The motivation for *The Practice of Electrocardiography* is to propose a solution for this enigma by describing the methods needed for analysis and synthesis, and standards for the product, a complete and adequate report. This approach is planned especially for medical students who want to build a firm base of understanding, for house officers, more advanced but still mystified by some of the literature and by discussions on rounds and at conferences, and for nurses, especially those in monitoring units, who may occasionally be confused by the nomenclature they must deal with. Cardiologists who interpret tracings for others and would like to review why they think what they think, and to write more convincing reports, will find some useful insights. EKG technicians, and those who teach them or are responsible for their work, should also find the book helpful, especially Chapter Six on technical methods.

What one gets from *The Practice of Electrocardiography* will depend on what is brought to it, and how the knowledge will be applied. The objective is understanding, not speed. Speed and confidence come with experience and cannot be acquired without time and effort.

Observation has taught that medical students like to get right to the point, to do something rather than talk about it, and this has dictated the organization of the subject matter. After the point of departure, and the end sought, have been established, the reader is asked follow the instructions in Chapter Two to interpret a tracing. This how-to chapter is, I believe, unique in the literature and, like instruction in physical diagnosis, concerned mostly with methods. It also contains references to other sections of the book where anatomic and physiologic principles, analytic methods as such, and pragmatic application are each considered, and where references to the underlying literature can be found.

For one interested in some depth, the discipline of electrocardiography is put in historic perspective, and several subjects not covered in most other texts are considered. The not-very-technical section on technical methods is included to call attention to that area as a major source of clinical problems, and to emphasize the importance of the technician. Doctors don't have to be skilled at recording tracings, but do need to know what happens inside each instrument in the system, and how it affects the result. And doctors should have recorded at least a few EKGs, in order to be able to recognize technical problems and tell the technician how to correct them.

The index has been planned to make it easy to locate information on almost any subject or problem likely to be encountered—by any name.

The views expressed have been developed with the help of many, many teachers, medical students, house officers, practicing physicians, technicians, and patients during twenty-five years of a practice limited to electrocardiography while teaching students and technicians. Dr. James R. Dawson was especially influential early in the development of my thought processes, Dr. John A. Gronvall contributed much time and advice in development of the original version of the text, and data accumulated during summer research projects by Drs. Michael W. Coleman, David B. McDaniel, and Andrew J. Myrick Jr. when they were medical students are included in the essay on the determinants of voltage. It is a pleasure to acknowledge the support of Drs. Harper K. Hellems, Patrick H. Lehan, Angel Markow, David H. Mulholland, John B. O'Connell, Kurt D. Olinde, Gaston Rodriguez, and Thomas N. Skelton, and the counsel of Dr. Julius M. Cruse and other faculty associates. The support and advice of Mr. Thomas Lanigan of Humana Press, and the patience of the staff of the Departments of Medical Illustration, Photography, and Computer Graphics at the University of Mississippi have been invaluable.

Thos. M. Blake, MD

Contents

ONE

Introduction

Experience with patients, doctors, medical students, and over a million electrocardiograms (EKGs) has shown two things: First, it is still true that many people are leading miserable and unnecessarily restricted lives because electrocardiography is not being used to its greatest advantage,[1,2] and second, this could be corrected easily. The plan of this book is to explain these views, and suggest that correction calls for nothing more than recognition that the standards for the practice of electrocardiography are the same as those for any other aspect of medicine.

The Problems

There seems to be embedded in the system the notion that all doctors should know how to interpret EKGs just as they should know how to diagnose pneumonia. Most don't, however, and some perceive this as weakness, although it really reflects professional responsibility; what the tracing "says" may be important, and they do not want to take chances. The perception of it as weakness is an artifact; the premise is not valid. Before they were expected to recognize pneumonia they were taught not only the anatomy, physiology, and pathology of the respiratory system but also how to distinguish normal from abnormal and interpret the findings, i.e., physical diagnosis. They were taught the scientific base for electrocardiography, too, and its nomenclature, but not its physical diagnosis, how to analyze and interpret a tracing themselves, or how to judge an interpretation written by someone else.

Standards for Electrocardiography

An important fact, often overlooked, is that there are, as yet, no "industry standards" for electrocardiography. There are guidelines for indications, multiple choice questions on Board examinations, and calls for supervised training, but no specific recommendations for methods of analysis or for criteria for completeness and adequacy of the product, and no requirement that findings and reasoning be documented. Often electrocardiography seems to be treated as a minor skill, mostly pattern recognition and rule application rather than problem solving. Permission for practice of all aspects of medicine rests finally with patients, and they trust their doctors. The MD, or DO, degree itself is supposed to ensure that the doctor will do no harm, and beyond this there are clear guidelines for evaluating competency in every field but one, electrocardiography. Anybody with a license to practice can sign EKG reports legally; the only authority needed is the permission of the hospital staff, and this is likely to be granted because of proficiency in related fields. The patient does not know the difference. Kindness and compassion, skill at physical diagnosis and cardiac catheterization, or having seen large numbers of tracings will not suffice. For the patient's own doctor to look at a tracing and get some benefit from it without recording his or her findings is one thing, but for the primary doctor to depend to a large extent on interpretation by another is a very different matter. Criteria for assessing qualification to interpret tracings for others are needed.

EKG Interpreter as Secondary Doctor

An electrocardiographer, like a radiologist or pathologist, is a secondary doctor who reports an interpretation of a specialized laboratory study to the primary doctor who requested it, not to the patient. It is easy for a primary doctor to understand a report of anatomic abnormality seen in X-rays and tissue sections, but the relevance to symptoms and signs of a diagram representing energy in space and time is harder to see. The tracing has no meaning at all until it is converted to words, and the words used are so well known that, as with the jargon of football or sex, to ask the meaning of something might seem to mark one as somehow deficient. The language seems to have taken on a life of its own, to have become confused with the substance it represents, the medium to have become the message, and much of it is not standard or logical and has little relevance to signs or symptoms.

The Abstract Nature of Electrocardiography

Electrocardiography is very abstract in most senses and of little interest to workers in other fields.[4] Its basis in anatomy, physiology, and physics is well founded, but in application it remains almost completely clinical and empirical. What the tracing represents is energy, and although energy is a concept used by everyone, it is hard to pin down—even when considered only within the anatomic and physiologic bounds of the heart, subjects about which much is known, and the problem is compounded by the fact that the trace reduces the information from all parts of the heart to a single point. The course of this point in space and time, projected on a framework of lines representing three dimensions, is an EKG. Think of the ball in a football game, a point moving in time and space and projected on a network of lines. Its position at any instant, like the position of the trace, is a result of all the forces in the system, not only the players on the field and the rules of the game but also emotions, the weather, and other variables, some of which are known and some not. The path it follows in a series of instants has meaning only if the observer knows the rules and is prepared to evaluate all the variables. Understanding the rules of the game, and the name and function of each player, is just as necessary in electrocardiography as in football.

Usefulness of an EKG

Usefulness to the patient is the only measure of the value of a tracing, and frequently this depends on how the interpretation is stated. Any finding, or combination of findings, can be interpreted in more than one way, and proof of what is "correct" is extremely limited by the need for complex techniques of study that are not applied very often,[57] and by the lack of standard, quantitative definitions and criteria for even such apparently obvious concepts as hypertrophy, dilatation, infarct, tachycardia, and ischemia. Proof of the presence or absence of some anatomic lesions, left bundle branch block, for instance, is difficult, and that of ones affecting only function, such as ventricular strain, metabolic imbalance, or drug effect, depends entirely on clinical judgment. Normal is difficult to define closely,[8–10] and there are wide intraobserver and interobserver variations.[11,12] Documentation of findings, and a precise report that makes clear the difference between what is seen and what it is interpreted to mean, are just as important in electrocardiography as in a physical examination.

The Wide Range of Normal

Most doctors never have an opportunity to become familiar with the wide range of normal of the several elements of an EKG, individually or in their many possible combinations. Experience with physical diagnosis in medical school and internship, shared by all doctors, ensures that a random blood pressure of 142/82 will not be interpreted as *prima facie* evidence of heart disease, but there is not a comparable base for evaluation of EKGs; the only tracings most see are from their own patients. Sometimes it seems to be assumed that any abnormality mentioned in an EKG report, no matter how tangentially, even just a computer readout, is related to the patient's complaints, or evidence of some hitherto unsuspected disease, when in fact it may have no clinical importance at all when seen in context. The risk to the patient is increased if it is not recognized that caveats such as "possible," or "cannot rule out," have the effect of removing any meaning from what follows. It has been noted that there is often an inverse relation between confidence in a laboratory procedure and experience with it.[3]

The problem was stated well by Dr. Frank Wilson:[1]

> We shall not attempt a long discussion of the present wretched state of electrocardiographic diagnosis or the misery attributable to it. The errors made in this field are due in large measure to the same human frailties that are responsible for errors in others, medical and non-medical. We wish, however, to make a few

comments which appear to us worthwhile. In our opinion, no physician should refer a patient to another for an electrocardiographic examination and report without giving the referee a resume of the data which he has collected (if he has any) nor without letting him know exactly what information the electrocardiographic examination is expected to yield.

We think also that there are altogether too many physicians who want to, and try to, read electrocardiograms, but are unwilling to go back to the fundamental principles upon which the interpretation of the electrocardiograms must be based. In our opinion, it is impossible to use diagnostic criteria intelligently unless they are fundamentally sound and the foundations on which they rest are clearly understood by the user.

Electrocardiography is one of the most exact of diagnostic methods. Its potential value is great, but it is not being used to the best advantage. Electrocardiographic abnormalities are not diseases. They have no important bearing upon life expectancy of the patient, or the extent to which his mode of life should be altered when there is reasonable doubt as to the nature of the factor or factors responsible for them in that particular case.

The same author observed later that the average American is at greater risk of being harmed by an EKG interpretation than by an atomic bomb.[935]

To summarize: Patients accept real risk in having an electrocardiogram made. They do not bleed, suffer physical pain, or die as a result of inadequate or inappropriate interpretation of tracings, but they often do suffer unnecessary anxiety, fiscal discomfort, problems with insurance programs and job security, and similar undesirable consequences, i.e., harm.

The Solution

The answer is to recognize interpretation of EKGs as the practice of medicine. The first rule for that, as everyone knows, is to do no harm, and there are two other rules for the practice of electrocardiography: first, define terms, and use the definitions consistently;

and second, be as specific as possible, and speculate beyond that to the degree appropriate, making clear where reporting ends and interpretation begins. Sometimes the findings in a tracing lead to a straightforward, uncontroversial answer, but often intuition and clinical experience are factors; the doctor must do the right thing, make decisions even when the data on which they must be based are incomplete, the decisions difficult, and the consequences considerable.[702]

It is easy to interpret EKGs, just as it is easy to practice neurosurgery or play the pipe organ, all one has to do is know how, but, in the case of electrocardiography, clear instructions for this have been hard to come by. Nobody would expect a medical student to go directly to ward work from the course in pathology, learning how to take a history and do a physical examination from attendance at rounds, and reading the current literature; but electrocardiography is often treated much this way, as something to be picked up along the way, and "brushed up" on later by taking a "refresher course."

Those who want to learn need instruction in the methods of the discipline: methods comparable to the vital signs, inspection, palpation, percussion, and auscultation of physical diagnosis. For electrocardiography, these are rates and intervals, orientation, duration, amplitude, and contour (Chapter Seven). The system and standards described in the following pages are based on these and can be useful not only for beginners but also for those charged with assessing competence. Every step in the process, from the time one first picks up a tracing until a complete and adequate report of what it says is ready to be signed, will be explained in detail.

There are two tools I can use to try to get these ideas across and convince you of their relevance and importance: words and pictures. The cliche that a picture is worth a thousand words is often applicable, but not always; to label a Q wave on a picture of an EKG is not much more instructive than to label a quarterback on a picture of a football team. Pictures, i.e., tracings and diagrams, are helpful and will be used, but the book should be thought of as a laboratory manual, not an atlas; the few tracings it contains are prototypes for reference; all were recorded at 25 mm/s and a standard of 1 mV producing a deflection of 10 mm. Words are the primary tool, and words are arbitrary; they depend for their effectiveness on agreement, agreement by all who use them as to their meanings. There is nothing inherently red about the word *red*, for instance; some other combination of letters could have the same significance, and indeed *rouge* does convey the same idea to millions who would not understand *red*, but so could *grandma*, or even *blue*.[920] For an adjective to work, the alternatives it excludes must be understood. In this exercise we assume standard English, of course, and, applying the rules strictly, this defines a problem immediately; most words have more than one meaning. In everyday discourse, speakers and hearers choose the right one intuitively in context, but in electrocardiography this is not always easy, and it is often not at all clear what is meant. If the doctor who performs and interprets a study is also the one who acts on it, as is usually the case with cardiac catheterization, for instance, and electrophysiologic studies, the written report of the procedure is for the record, off line. In electrocardiography, though, the report is on line, between the doctor who writes it and the patient. Its effect will depend on what the doctor who reads it perceives it to mean. Those who write such reports are responsible for expressing themselves clearly, and this is made difficult by the custom of using a jargon full of opaque terms, some of which have been in use nearly a hundred years and do not have the same meaning as when they were introduced. The goal is not (necessarily) to change the language, but to provide insight into the limitations it imposes, and due regard for the need for precision.[13]

Within the small discipline we are concerned with now, we must try hard to have only *one meaning for each word/symbol*. This requires effort. The use of words from the common language, whose meaning is clear to laymen as well as doctors, to imply something different in the (pseudo)scientific jargon of electrocardiography introduces unnecessary problems and is to be avoided whenever possible; *rhythm* is such a word (*see* Appendix). The definitions that follow are proposed as a beginning. For the most part, they are not controversial, but they do not have the weight of law, or even tradition in some cases; their usefulness depends on your acceptance of them as having "the ring of truth." The unique feature of this collection is that they are documented and can be used as a stable foundation. Read them and think about them, but do not spend much time on any one, or try to memorize anything. The object of this first contact is to become aware that there is a firm base, that there are definitions to which you can refer. Watch for times when they shed light on what is happening as you analyze and interpret tracings. If in your judgment one is not valid, or does not apply to you, note this, record your alternative, and observe the effects of the change on the decision-making process. The intent is to work from the inside out, internal electrocardiography in the same sense that we speak of internal medicine,[913] from the ground up, not just to present the view from the outside with labels on things. Patterns count, but understanding how they got that way enhances their usefulness and contributes to confidence.

Definitions

The EKG vocabulary known by all doctors has been in place for a long time and is not often questioned, but the implications of many of its accepted terms are far from clear, a situation that limits the usefulness of the method and puts the patient at unnecessary risk. The following definitions will be used consistently in this book, and other key words are discussed in the Appendix.

The Tracing and Its Components

1. **Electrocardiogram (EKG or ECG):** A graphic representation of the electrical activity of the heart in a series of beats; specifically, a record of the course through space of the net result of this activity, a single point (A), as it departs from a fixed point (B) in the center of the chest and returns to it.

    The unit of the system, the record of a single cardiac cycle, consists of a family of curves known as P, Q, R, S, T, and U.

2. **B point:** The central reference point for electrocardiography, represented in the tracing by the point of junction of PQ and QRS, the beginning of the QRS complex, the base point.

    Atrial repolarization is in progress here, and the U-P segment is nearer to the theoretical level of zero potential, but U-P is often unstable and hard to define. Atrial repolariza-

tion is a negligible factor in the surface tracing, and the B
point is the most reproducible base, the graphic equivalent
of Einthoven's single dipole, Wilson's central terminal of
zero potential, the middle of the fifty yard line. Everything
in the tracing is measured to it, from it, above it, or below it
(*see* Ground, in Appendix).

3. **Baseline:** A line connecting the B points of two contiguous
   beats in as nearly flat a section of the lead as possible.

   The baseline should be defined as the level of the trace
   when there is no electrical activity. Theoretically, this means
   the UP segment, and when the trace is stable and flat, the UP
   and PQ segments, J, and the tiny segment between T and U,
   are all at the same level. This is not true, however, when there is
   muscle tremor, atrial fibrillation or flutter, P is too small to
   define clearly, or when the level of the trace varies because
   electrodes are not snugly applied. The baseline is especially
   likely to be unstable in tracings made during or immediately
   after exercise when its definition is critical. Pragmatically,
   the B point (above) is the most stable point in the tracing. A
   horizontal line through a single B point is not enough to define
   the baseline; it takes two points to determine a line.

4. **J point:** The junction of QRS and ST.

   J is really a small area, a shoulder, rather than a literal
   point, and defining it calls for judgment. Its position with
   relation to the baseline defines orientation and amplitude of
   the forces that write ST; e.g., up in Lead I and down in aVF
   and V1 means orientation to the left, up, and dorsad. To define
   departure of the trace from the baseline as elevation or depression requires that the lead be named; the generic designation
   is *displacement*. There is only one PQRSTU; the tracing
   shows it in three dimensions, information in any lead is the
   same as that all other leads, only the view varies.

5. **Deflection/wave:** Excursion of the trace above or below the
   baseline is a deflection; return to the baseline completes a wave.

   In practice, the two words are used almost synonymously.
   There may be notches in a wave but it is not complete until it
   returns to the baseline.

6. **P:** A small wave (compared to QRS), the first wave generated in a normal heartbeat.

   It is discrete, recurrent (except in the case of premature
   atrial beats, "PACs"), and represents excitation of the atria
   in a coordinated fashion. In the normal heart it follows discharge of the sinus node and is directed leftward, downward,
   and initially ventrad and terminally dorsad. Of these directions, the downward (caudad) one is most important. If it
   arises outside the sinus node, its orientation and contour are
   modified accordingly and it is said to be of ectopic origin.
   To identify a wave as a "P" is to say that the atria are being
   depolarized in an organized fashion, but it does not imply
   sinus origin.

   Sometimes a P wave thought to have originated outside the
   sinus node is identified as P'. This is in conflict with the definition given here in that it substitutes interpretation for description and uses the prime mark for a purpose other than the more
   traditional one of designating repeated waves, e.g., RSR'.
7. **PR interval:** The time from the beginning of P to the beginning of QRS, whether the initial deflection in the QRS is
   positive or negative; it may really be a PQ interval.
8. **PQ segment:** That section of the trace between the end of P
   and the beginning of QRS.
9. **f waves:** Completely irregular undulation of the baseline,
   typical of random electrical activity of muscle fibers or fascicles, chaos as distinguished from organized activity, but
   typically of lower frequency than the chaos of skeletal muscle
   activity with which they may be confused.

   f waves define atrial fibrillation. *See* P wave.
10. **QRS:** The combination of waves written by depolarization
    of the ventricles, typically three but there may be any number.

    The complex is known generically as a QRS no matter
    what its specific components.
11. **Q wave:** A negative wave that initiates the QRS and is fol-
    lowed by an R wave.
12. **R wave:** Any positive wave in the QRS; more than one, R',
    R", etc.

13. **S wave:** Any negative wave in the QRS following an R wave; more than one, S', S'', etc.
14. **QS:** A completely negative QRS complex.
15. **T wave:** A long, slow wave following QRS.

    It is attributable to ventricular repolarization and is subdivided into an early, basically horizontal component, the ST segment, and a terminal, basically vertical one, the T wave. The designation "T" is used sometimes to refer to the whole curve, and sometimes only the terminal part of it selectively. *See* ST-T.
16. **ST-T:** A term that emphasizes reference to the whole curve of ventricular repolarization, both ST and T, the ST-T complex.
17. **QT interval:** The time from the beginning of QRS to the end of T.

    QT is a measure of the duration of ventricular repolarization, *electrical systole*; QRS coincides with the first heart sound, the return stroke of T with the second. Repolarization is assumed to begin at the same time as depolarization; QRS is inscribed during QT.
18. **U wave:** A small, slow wave that follows T, usually seen best in a right precordial lead.

    It is probably related to ventricular repolarization, but delayed potentials from depolarization may be a factor. It is not identifiable in every tracing.
19. **Wave:** A round trip of the trace from baseline to baseline. *See* Deflection above.

Technical Features of the Tracing

20. **Format:** The order in which the leads are presented.

    There is no single right or wrong format, and one must be alert for different ones. The most common one in current use displays 12 leads in three channels recorded simultaneously, four groups of 2.5 s each; the first group is leads I, II, and III (from top to bottom) followed by aVR-aVL-aVF, V1-V2-V3, and V4-V5-V6. In most, but not all, formats, time is continuous across lead changes, and leads are labeled or coded.

21. **Calibration:** A record of the amplitude of the deflection pro-
    duced by 1 mV, of the frequency response of the recording
    system, and, in most current EKG machines, of paper speed.

    All vertical measurements in the tracing are referred to a
    standard: 1 mV = 10 mm. In automatically calibrated equip-
    ment, the millivolt signal lasts 0.20 s and its width docu-
    ments the paper speed: 5 mm, 25 mm/s; 10 mm, 50 mm/s.

22. **Paper speed:** The EKG chart consists of horizontal and ver-
    tical lines at 1 mm intervals with each fifth one accentuated.
    For 1 mm to represent 0.04 s the paper must move at exactly
    25 mm/s, and this is standard.

    The only problem likely to occur results from paper speed
    50 mm/s, which makes the interval 0.02 s. The way to check
    this on modern machines is at the calibration mark. *See*
    Calibration.

See Appendix for other critical words and phrases.

TWO

How to Describe and Interpret an Electrocardiogram

Sir William Osler noted that the most efficient way to utilize one's gifts with the least possible effort is to cultivate system,[916] and system is so basic to the way doctors think most of the time that they are hardly even aware of it. The order for taking a history and doing a physical examination, for instance, for documenting the findings and recording a diagnosis, is universal. The purpose of this chapter is to describe a similar approach to electrocardiograms.

Observation and explanation are separate processes by definition, but distinction between them blurs during the acquisition of data, in electrocardiography as in physical examination. To describe an abnormal Q wave without being aware of ST elevation in the same lead, and suspecting that they are related, is no more possible, or necessary, than to describe a murmur without being alert to the râles and edema that are inescapably apparent at the same time, and recognizing that they are probably parts of the same problem; nevertheless, it is important to distinguish between objectively demonstrable individual findings and subjective evaluation of what they mean. The difference between analysis and synthesis is recognized routinely in physical examination, the diagnosis is not recorded until the findings leading to it have been documented, and the same approach can be applied in examination of an electrocardiogram. The worksheet shown in Fig. 2-1 is a framework for this process. As with the more familiar order for the physical examination, it is not only a guide for the systematic acquisition of data, but also a vehicle for their display and evaluation, a means to an end.

The text of this chapter follows the order of the worksheet, giving instructions for describing each element of the tracing. Its format is planned to facilitate rapid alternation between description and interpretation without losing sight of the difference, suggesting

13

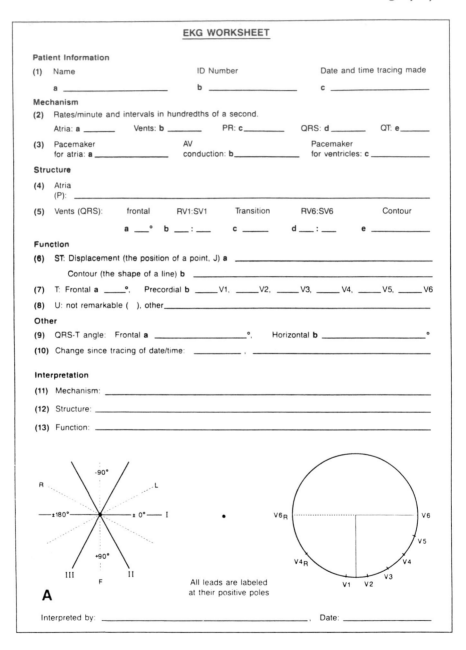

EKG WORKSHEET

Patient Information

(1) Name   ID Number   Date and time tracing made

    a _____   b _____   c _____

Mechanism

(2) Rates/minute and intervals in hundredths of a second.

    Atria: a _____   Vents: b _____   PR: c_____   QRS: d _____   QT: e_____

(3) Pacemaker   AV   Pacemaker
    for atria: a _____   conduction: b_____   for ventricles: c _____

Structure

(4) Atria
    (P): _____

(5) Vents (QRS):   frontal   RV1:SV1   Transition   RV6:SV6   Contour

    a ___° b ___ : ___   c _____   d ___ : ___   e _____

Function

(6) ST: Displacement (the position of a point, J) a _____

    Contour (the shape of a line) b _____

(7) T: Frontal a _____°,   Precordial b _____V1, _____V2, _____V3, _____V4, _____V5, _____V6

(8) U: not remarkable ( ), other_____

Other

(9) QRS-T angle: Frontal a _____°,   Horizontal b _____°

(10) Change since tracing of date/time: _____ , _____

Interpretation

(11) Mechanism: _____

(12) Structure: _____

(13) Function: _____

All leads are labeled
at their positive poles

A

Interpreted by: _____ , Date: _____

Fig. 2-1. Worksheet.

in inset paragraphs the interpretation appropriate at each stage. There are frequent references to other sections of the book, where more information is available and access to the literature is provided, and at the end there is a discussion of the kinds of thinking involved in rearrangement of data into a useful interpretation. When all the steps have been practiced a few times, the order for study of an EKG can be as integral a part of one's "system" as that for the history or physical examination, not something memorized, not an imposed chore, but a convenient statement of the way things are.

How to Use This Book

Most readers will be familiar already with the basic nomenclature of the electrocardiogram described in the definitions (p. 8) and illustrated in Fig. 2-2. Assuming this, you are ready to begin to work with real tracings. The book is organized with the idea of electrocardiography as a continuous process, with the patient as its origin and termination, a loop that should be closed. Beginning with definitions, it proceeds through a summary of the anatomy and physiology represented in the tracing, the equipment used, and the role of the technicians who operate it, the methods of analysis and interpretation, and ending with communication between the doctor responsible for production and interpretation and the one who ordered the study and will use the information it yields in making decisions that will affect the patient.

The recommended approach is to use Chapter Two as a dissection manual. Reproduce the worksheet (the one at the back of the book is suitable for photocopying) and follow the instructions, filling out *every* blank. DO NOT spend time reviewing your Physiology notes now. They will be helpful after a problem has been identified, but at this point the object is to identify the problem and name it. Scan the chapter if you wish, but DO NOT try to read it through and then try to apply it; that would be no more logical than it would have been to read your physical diagnosis book and then take a history and do a physical examination. Take *one step at time*. The chapter is long, and can be tedious at first, just as the writeup of your first history

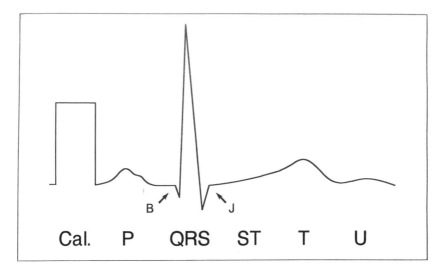

Fig. 2-2. The unit of the EKG.

and physical was. If you get tired or impatient, stop. Come back to it later. The second time around, it will go faster and make more sense. Don't push yourself, take as many sessions as you need, but commit yourself to make a decision about the information called for in each space. If it isn't available, or relevant, or you don't understand the question, enter a dash. If you aren't sure, ask for help, the index is a good source; if it still isn't clear, enter a question mark. An empty space may mean the information was not available, that you did not know the answer, or that you overlooked that point, but a dash or a question mark shows someone reviewing your work where you need help. When an entry is outside the limits of normal, mark it for later consideration.

Every effort has been made to give all the instruction needed, but some test of the result is a necessity. Primary practitioners get instant and effective feedback from their patients, but electrocardiographers, who report to other doctors, rarely know what effect their efforts produce, and must be especially mindful that what they report is accurate the first time. One safeguard is to check your work the same way you check addition or subtraction; be sure that each of the abnormalities marked during description is accounted for in the interpretation, and that each component of the interpretation is justified in the description. The ultimate test of whether your interpretation is right or wrong is its effect on the patient, but this requires that you know the whole clinical picture, and this is not always possible. The tutorial support of an experienced practitioner is still needed, but for this to be effective it must be specific. To be told that a finding has a certain significance, without being told precisely how that is known, is not enough.

Collateral reading in other texts, especially the original literature, will be helpful. All books have something to offer, some students learn better from one teacher than another, and often a point is clearer the second time around.

Patient Identification

Line 1

Unidentified data are useless at best, and potentially hazardous. Name, number, date, and time are all important.

> Identification of the patient is critical; to compare tracings from different people, or to attribute findings in a tracing to the wrong patient, can have dire consequences. Both number and name are needed, the number serving as a double check; there may be other people with the same name, but there should not be anybody else with the same number. The date and time the tracing was made can be crucial.

Mechanism

Line 2

2a. Atrial rate. The first blank calls for atrial rate, and, because the atria are almost always activated before the ventricles, this is the proper place to display it, but in practice the first thing measured is ventricular rate. Atrial rate will be discussed below at the proper time.

2b. Ventricular rate. All EKG paper is ruled with horizontal and vertical lines at one millimeter intervals, every fifth one accentuated, but formats for display and labeling of leads, and for marking lead changes, are not standard. In some systems, paper transport is not continuous. Be sure of the features of your tracing (p. 11).

Three-cycle-length and two-cycle-length ratemeters, readily available from manufacturers of EKG equipment, have about the same credibility as the common practice of estimating the heart rate by counting the pulse for 15 s and multiplying by four. In the absence of a ratemeter, the vertical marks in the margins of some EKG paper represent 3 s, and it is easy to count across two of these and multiply by ten; to divide one cycle length into 60 s is useful but assumes a perfectly regular rhythm. Enter the figure for ventricular rate in the spaces for both atria (2a) and ventricles (2b), assuming for the time being that they are the same. If they are not, or if there are no P waves, this will become apparent when it is time to estimate the PR interval, and the figure for atrial rate can be changed.

Rates cannot be estimated usefully any more closely by electrocardiography than by physical examination, and to distinguish between 81 and 82 beats per minute as if the difference were meaningful is a mistake; about five beats per minute is a reasonable limit of the method for rates between 50 and 100, closer than that at very slow rates, and less at very rapid ones. Atrial and ventricular rates may not be the same.

There is no blank on the worksheet for the rhythm of either atria or ventricles, but there is plenty of space in the margins for comment; if there is no note to the contrary, it will be assumed to be approximately regular (*see sinus arrhythmia*, p. 123).

Ventricular rates between 40 and 140 can be presumed to represent sinus origin if the rhythm is regular, and atrial fibrillation if it is irregular, until proved otherwise. Rates below forty raise the question of AV block (p. 150). Ventricular rates above 160 are unusual with sinus mechanism (except when there is an obvious explanation, such as impairment of oxygen transfer) but are typical with usurping ectopy. Between 140 and 160, no matter what the rhythm, there is a good chance that there is atrial ectopy at a rate of around 300 with second degree AV block; look carefully for extra Ps, and read about atrial flutter (p. 129).

2a. Atrial rate (moved from above). The next blank is for the PR interval, and, if atrial rate is the same as ventricular, all that is needed to determine it is to measure the time from the beginning of P to the beginning of QRS. The figure that was entered for atrial rate was really for the ventricles, though, and now is the time to check it, to identify atrial activity. What to expect has been suggested already by the ventricular rate and rhythm; there only two common chronic forms of atrial activity, sinus and fibrillation. Distinction between them on physical examination depends mainly on their effect on ventricular rhythm, but in the electrocardiogram atrial and ventricular signals can be separated and atrial activity examined directly without regard for its effect on the ventricles. If atrial complexes are very small, however, or if atria and ventricles are generating information at the same time, this may not be possible.

First, is there atrial activity, any fluctuation of the trace between QRSs (other than T and U waves and isolated premature beats)? If there is, it is either repetitive and discrete or continuous and irregular, predictable or unpredictable, P waves or fibrillary waves. *P waves* mean that the atria are being depolarized in an organized fashion. Their rate should be recorded in 2a, replacing the figure already there if necessary. It may be anywhere from below 30 to over 200, and it may not be the same as ventricular rate. If there is *atrial fibrillation*, enter a dash in 2a and write AF in space 3a and on Line Eleven. If no atrial activity is visible (p. 122), enter a dash in 2a and 3a; a name for the mechanism, to be entered on Line Eleven, will be considered later.

The presence of P waves eliminates atrial standstill (p. 123), atrial fibrillation, and a midjunctional mechanism from consideration but does not by itself identify a sinus origin; P waves may arise in the sinus node, anywhere in either atrium, or even below the AV node. The means for determining their point of origin will be discussed on Line Three, and their morphology is considered on Line Four, but for now the only question is whether there are P waves, and the features most critical in defining that are the discrete nature and predictable recurrence of small waves. Isolated, premature beats (PACs, *see* p. 127) are an exception.

Atrial fibrillation is recognized by wiggly undulation of the baseline; nothing is repetitive (p. 131). It may be very coarse, or so fine that it is hardly detectable, and may be simulated closely by muscle tremor (p. 102). It is just as true in the EKG as on physical examination that ventricular rhythm is typically irregularly irregular when there is atrial fibrillation, and, when atrial activity is not clear, the QRS rhythm is helpful in making a decision, but when the ventricular rate is very rapid or very slow, irregularity of its rhythm may not be obvious. Also, atrial fibrillation may be present even though, for one reason or another, ventricular rhythm is regular (p. 132).

If no atrial activity is identifiable but ventricular rhythm is regular, there may be sinus activity with P waves too small to see, a midjunctional pacemaker, or some other explanation (p. 122). If ventricular rhythm is grossly irregular, there is probably atrial fibrillation, but other explanations are possible e.g., sinus mechanism with PACs. When atrial activity is not visible, professional judgment is required for determining whether it is absent or just too small to see, and must take into account all the information available. This not an unusual problem, especially when the baseline is unstable, when there is muscle tremor artifact, and in old people.

2c. PR. Horizontal measurements in the trace represent time and vary inversely with the rate. They are estimated in the lead in which they are longest *and* can be determined with the greatest confidence—two criteria, sometimes not both fulfilled in the same lead, posing a small problem. There is a temptation to feel that the closer an interval is called, the more precise the analysis, but the limits of the method must be respected. There is real danger that more significance may be attached to such "precision" than it merits, and this can work to the patient's disadvantage. Knowing for oneself what is meaningful and what is not is important and depends on informed experience in a clinical context.

The PR interval is measured from the beginning of P to the beginning of QRS and represents the time required for the excitation process to go from the sinus node to the ventricles; the accuracy with which it can be measured is limited by the fact that it is hard to be sure just where P begins. Choose a point and estimate the time from it to the B point. To enter a figure for PR is to say that the same impulse responsible for atrial activity traversed the AV junction and gave rise to ventricular activity. If atrial and ventricular rates are not the same, or even if they are the same but there is atrial tachycardia or flutter, no PR interval should be indicated; a dash goes in 2c.

In most adults, PR is about 0.16 to 0.20 s. 0.12 is not unusual at rapid rates (>100), and 0.24 is borderline at slow ones (<50). It can be measured usefully no closer than 0.04 s. No lower limit of normal can be set.

Medical students seem to learn early that the "upper limit of normal" for PR is 0.20 s, and that values higher than this define first degree AV block (p. 150). A good figure to remember is 0.20, but as the usual one for adults, not the upper limit of normal, a number comparable to 120 for systolic blood pressure. Some, who recognize their own limitations in measuring PR, assume that the computer can accomplish the task unerringly and to the millisecond, but this is not true; it can do only what it is been programmed to do. It can be trusted to bring exactly the same standards to bear every time, but depends on human ability to tell it where P begins—and this is limited.

When there is doubt about whether PR is long, it is not. A value of 0.28 or greater is first degree AV block no matter what the rate, but what it means to the patient must be determined in the context of many factors, including its stability; 0.24 calls for judgment. First degree AV block is not a disease but simply a name for a finding in a tracing. It does not necessarily predict greater degrees of block (p. 151).

AV block is often called "heart block," but that's not being as precise as the method allows. Intraventricular block is also "heart" block, and the patient, who may hear the words, and who knows the heart is a pump, may think of mechanical obstruction. A diagnosis of "heart block" is sometimes assumed to identify pathology when what it really represents is only someone's estimate of where the P begins—to a quarter of a millimeter—and this is meaningless. PR can be too short, just as the blood pressure can be too low, or the white count or the temperature, but no lower limit can be defined arbitrarily; other factors must be taken into account. It is short with ventricular pre-excitation, the "WPW syndrome," but this is secondary to excitation of the ventricles prematurely via an anomalous pathway that conducts more rapidly than the AV node, not a greater rate of conduction through normal AV pathways; the primary abnormality is recognized in the early part of the QRS (p. 155). The Lown–Ganong–Levine syndrome is a clinical diagnosis of which a short PR is a part (p. 157).

2d. QRS. The duration of QRS is the time elapsed between B and J, but, as with the beginning of P, J is hard to pin down precisely. Following the rule that duration is estimated in the lead in which it is longest *and* can be defined satisfactorily, it is usually measured in a right precordial lead, despite the fact that the end of QRS is particularly hard to localize there. Recognizing this problem, it is wiser to call it too narrow than too wide when there is doubt. At a clinically useful level, the decision is simply whether it is *wide* or *not wide*, based on inspection, and the perception of contour as normal or not is undoubtedly a subliminal factor in this decision. The conclusion is expressed in numbers, but they represent practiced judgment, not precise measurement. Computer programmers have done a remarkable job of simulating this process but have not yet duplicated it.

QRS duration is about 0.06 s to 0.08 s in the usual adult, as brief as 0.04 in infants, and 0.10 is the time-honored upper limit of normal, seen commonly in the elderly. The limit of the method is 0.02 s.

Ventricular depolarization may be slowed by various means, but can't be speeded up beyond normal; QRS can be too wide but not too narrow. If it is not clear whether it is wide or not, look at examples of some that are obviously wide; PVCs (Fig. 8-6), for instance, or bundle branch block (Figs. 10-1 and 10-2). If it still is not clear, call it 0.10 s. A figure of 0.12 or greater means it is wide and must be accounted for in the interpretation on Line Twelve. There is almost always some slurring or notching of complexes that are truly wide.

The tendency of beginners is to measure QRS duration with calipers with the intent of objective accuracy, but this is like reading a sphygmomanometer with a magnifying lens; it is better to estimate it by inspection with the aid of only the millimeter grid on the paper. The end point, J, is difficult to define very precisely, and the range of normal is wide. Computer programs are likely to call QRS duration longer than it should be called. When this happens, and no explanation for widening is apparent in other parameters as programmed, especially contour, the readout will either fail to note it or will mark it by some expression such as "atypical intraventricular conduction delay," bringing it to the attention of the interpreter for a decision. Artifactual widening is sometimes the result of merging of QRS with atrial activity, especially when there is atrial flutter, so that a P is perceived as a Q, an R, or an S. Whether it is really wide, and if so what the widening means, is a decision to be made by a human. Prolongation is usually associated with abnormality of contour (space 5e). The computer, like a lawn mower or a scalpel, works for the user, not the other way around (p. 224).

2e. QT. The duration of the QT interval represents the time required for ventricular repolarization. This starts before depolarization has been completed, and, because the trace represents both processes, and the precise instant during the QRS at which recovery begins cannot be pinpointed, it is assumed to begin at the same time as QRS. QT is measured from the B point to the end of T. The first heart sound coincides with QRS, the second with the return stroke of T, and QT has been called "electrical systole."

In adults, most QT intervals fall between 0.32 and 0.44 s, with 0.36 or 0.40 s the usual value. A figure greater than 0.44 almost always represents inclusion of the U wave. It cannot be estimated usefully any closer than 0.04 s. Sometimes confident distinction between T and U is not possible, and, when merging of the two is suspected, it can often be demonstrated by a "dimple" where they meet, usually seen best in a right precordial lead (p. 217).

Change in QT is very nonspecific, not only because of the limits of the method for determining just where T ends, but also because almost any change that affects it makes it longer— almost, but not all (p. 202). The practice of calculating a "QTc," or "corrected QT," a single figure incorporating both the measured QT and the rate, makes sense but has very limited value. There is no doubt that the interval varies inversely with the rate, but to "correct" such an inherently imprecise value by mathematical manipulation, especially when even the "corrected" number means so little, is not very productive. *See* page 202 for further discussion of QT and the problem of its accurate estimation.

Line 3

With the first two lines finished, most of the information needed to name the mechanism is available, and will be developed further on Line Three. Nowhere in electrocardiography is the terminology more confusing than here, especially failure to distinguish between what is seen and what it is thought to mean. Using the definitions in the Appendix, though, it is possible to arrive at a useful statement that will tell another doctor the location of the pacemaker for the atria, its rate and rhythm, the same for the ventricles, and the causal relation, if any, between the two systems. An explanation for the findings, what normal or pathologic processes they reflect, especially the means by which a usurping mechanism is sustained, is a different subject that requires judgment based on the most plausible current thinking (*see* Chapter Eight). The common practice of offering an explanation for the problem without naming it is in conflict with the second rule, to be as specific as possible; speculating beyond that is a separate step (p. 6), and sometimes mystifies more than it demystifies. What the tracing shows is one thing; how it got that way is something else. Sir James Mackenzie noted in 1925 that

"One should be chary of inventing new names or of altering old ones, for the name usually represents the imperfect knowledge at the moment it is given."[917]

3a. Pacemaker for atria. Atrial rate and rhythm have been noted already. Further information about atrial activity is needed before it can be evaluated completely, and instruction for this will be given below, but in practice the ventricular complex is considered first.

3b. Relation between atrial and ventricular activity. This cannot be determined until each has been considered separately, and the ventricles are usually analyzed first.

3c. Pacemaker for the ventricles. What is *known* about the origin of the impulse that depolarizes the ventricles? In most cases the answer is clear from the figure recorded for QRS duration in 2d; if that figure is not greater than 0.10, the rate of propagation through the His–Purkinje system and myocardium has been as rapid as possible (p. 76), i.e, normal. If QRS is *not wide*, then, the impulse for depolarization must have entered the ventricles from some point proximal to the bifurcation of the Bundle of His; i.e., it is of supraventricular origin. Localization of the site precisely will be discussed next, but the only question now is whether it is above the bifurcation of the bundle of His or below it.

A wide QRS may mean that the beat originated in the ventricular wall, whether as an isolated event (a PVC, *see* p. 142), repetitively at a slow rate (as with a default pacemaker compensating for third-degree AV block, *see* p. 140), a rapid one (ventricular tachycardia, *see* p. 144), or in between (p. 145), but it may also represent an intraventricular conduction defect in a beat of supraventricular origin.

Very commonly, medical students enter "supraventricular" in space 3c, and, when asked to explain how they know that, say it is because there is a P before each QRS. That is the wrong answer. P represents atrial activity, and the subject now is ventricular activity. It's true that there is a 1:1 relation between Ps and QRSs in an uncomplicated sinus mechanism, but other explanations for a 1:1 ratio are possible (pp. 129,

131, 134). The fact that QRS is *not wide* is what identifies it as of supraventricular origin, not its relation to atrial activity.

For present purposes it is assumed that the QRS is not wide; "supraventricular" goes in 3c.

3a. Pacemaker for the atria (moved from above). Next, what is driving the atria? There are several loci north of the bifurcation of the Bundle of His that have the capacity for initiating impulses, and the active one must be identified as closely as possible. Knowing the rate and rhythm of the ventricles, and that they are activated from above, gives one a pretty good idea of what is going on in the "supraventricles," and the figures on Line Two will have suggested this already. If there is no atrial activity, or if there is atrial fibrillation, this will have been noted; for present purposes it is assumed that there are P waves. The question now is their origin, and the most important indicators of this are their orientation and whether they precede or follow QRS.

A normal P wave originates in the *sinus node* and is directed to the left (positive in Lead I), caudad (positive in aVF), and initially ventrad and terminally dorsad (initially positive and terminally negative in V1). Any other point of origin is ectopic, and there are several possibilities. An impulse that arises in tissue just above the AV node (*high junctional*, low atrial) spreads over the atria retrograde, producing a P wave that precedes QRS, is negative in leads II, III, and aVF, and often V-shaped; one from below the AV node (*low junctional* or His bundle, or a *ventricle*), a similar retrograde P, but following QRS (p. 126). If the origin is not clear, but thought not to be sinus, it is called just *atrial*. P wave morphology is considered in more detail on Line Four.

3b. Relation between atria and ventricles (PR). Having identified the pacemaker for the atria, that for the ventricles, and the rate and rhythm of each, the next step is to assess the causal relation between them, if any (not counting PACs and PVCs). If atrial and ventricular rates are the same, one option is to write "normal" in this space. That makes sense, but is an interpretation; a more objective observation would be "1:1"; the judgment that this is normal will be implicit in the statement of the mechanism, and in most cases the following brief instructions will lead to a satisfactory designation of this. If atrial and ventricular rates are not the same, or even if they are but P is not of sinus origin, put a dash in the space for PR.

If there is a P, it's directed to the left and/or caudad, its rate is between about 40 and 140, its rhythm is approximately regular, and it occurs in a 1:1 ratio to QRS, the mechanism is *sinus*. If PR is long, 0.28 s or more, there is first degree *AV block* (p. 150); if the P:QRS ratio is not 1:1 and QRS is slower than P, there is second- or third-degree AV block (*see* p. 121 for the image of the atria as a funnel); if QRS is faster, two foci are active (pp. 133, 144). If the rate of P is above about 150 and not clearly of sinus origin (*see* 3a), read about usurping atrial ectopy (p. 127). If the trace shows irregular fluctuation between ventricular complexes, there is atrial fibrillation. Premature beats are common. If they are not preceded by Ps, and their QRS is different from others in the same lead and clearly wide, they are probably of ventricular origin, PVCs (p. 142), but may be supraventricular with aberration (p. 169); if of the same duration and configuration as in other beats in the same lead, supraventricular, called *PAC*s even though it may not be possible to identify a P before each one, (p. 127).

These instructions are intended for beginners and are not detailed enough for complicated disorders of impulse formation and/or conduction. If what is happening in the atria and ventricles in a series of beats seems understandable at this point, that's enough. Mechanism disorders are discussed in more detail in Chapters Eight and Nine.

Structure

Line 4

Atria: P wave. P waves should be described clearly enough to establish credibility, but it is often difficult to know exactly how to do this. Their most important feature is simply their presence, and the principal marker of this, when all arise from the same focus, is the predictable recurrence of small waves (but with isolated beats, PACs, even this criterion does not apply). They are usually seen best in Leads II, III, aVF, and/or V1, but the lead in which they are seen is irrelevant, and they may be so small that quantitative description of neither orientation, duration, amplitude, or contour is practical.

The *normal P* is small compared to QRS in the same lead, sometimes so small that judgment is necessary to be sure about it, but usually large enough to be seen easily. Its most important feature other than repetitiveness, is its *orientation*. The reference frames used for this are shown at the bottom of the worksheet, and their derivation is discussed in Chapter Five. Detailed instruction for determination of orientation is given under description of QRS in Line Five, and is equally applicable to all elements of the tracing, but, for now, orientation of P can be handled simplistically. As the process of depolarization passes from the sinus node to the AV node, it produces a wave directed chiefly caudad, usually to the left, and initially ventrad and terminally dorsad; i.e., it is positive in Lead aVF, usually positive in Lead I, and initially positive and terminally negative in V1. The most consistent and important of these is its caudal direction. It is nearly always negative in aVR and terminally negative in V1, and this may be an important thing to know when mislabeling of leads is suspected (p. 104). Considering the limits imposed by the slow beginning and ending of P, and its relatively low voltage and small area, its *duration* is not useful information. The same is true of *amplitude* in any quantitative sense; it can be described as simply normal, low, tall, or deep, small, or prominent (compared to QRS)—judgment calls, but not difficult with a little experience. Note that these adjectives indicate, not only amplitude, but also orientation. For a wave to be described as "tall," the lead must be specified; what is tall in one view is deep from the opposite side and flat from halfway between. The *contour* of a normal P wave of sinus origin is usually a little rounded, and slightly notched just past its peak, especially in Lead II, but these features are subject to wide variation. The notch in Lead II, and change from initial positivity to terminal negativity in V1, reflect the passage of excitation from right atrium to left.

The origin of P is determined from the direction in which it is inscribed. A locus near the caudal end of an atrium produces retrograde depolarization of the atria, and a P that is negative in Leads II, III, and aVF; at the cephalic end, a P that may not be distinguishable from one of sinus origin; if the impulse arises in the midsection, its P may not be visible.

The only common abnormalities of P, other than orientation, are those of size and contour representing enlargement of either right and/or left atrium, each of which can be identified without regard to the other because, in contrast to the ventricles, which depolarize simultaneously, the atria depolarize sequentially, right followed by left. It was recognized early that a prominent, broad P in Lead II, with accentuation of the notch, correlates with *left atrial enlargement* and is seen commonly with mitral valve disease (p. 188). Prominence of the first part of the wave with diminution of the notch, leading to a smooth, tent-shaped contour, also seen best in Lead II, correlates with *right atrial enlargement* and is seen most commonly in patients with lung disease (p. 188). These classic observations are still valid, but prominence of the terminally negative component of P in V1 is a better indication of left atrial enlargement than the picture in Lead II; note that *prominence* is the key word, not just negativity, and *enlargement*, not hypertrophy or dilatation. The patterns were known originally as "P mitrale" and "P pulmonale," but these terms are used rarely now.

Before enlargement of either atrium is diagnosed, examples should be reviewed for perspective (Figs. 12-1 and 12-2). The range of normal is wide, and the tendency of some computer programs to overdiagnose left atrial enlargement and underdiagnose right should be recognized. Either is a real, anatomic abnormality that reflects real response to a real hemodynamic lesion, and must not be treated lightly, but at the same time distinction of either from normal may not be possible, and lack of evidence of either by no means "rules it out."

Line 5

Ventricles. Up to this point, analysis has consisted mostly of measuring rates and intervals, and noting the relatively simple patterns of atrial depolarization. The QRS is more complex, and the relevance of all four measurements, orientation, duration, amplitude, and contour, is obvious. It is the most stable part of the tracing, and, with the exception of drug effects, electrolyte imbalance, and a few other circumstances, abnormality here correlates with structural abnormality of the ventricular wall.

The QRS is a record of electrical forces, and any force has three properties, magnitude, sense, and direction. These can be represented by a line whose length is proportional to the strength of the force and whose orientation in space is the same as that of the force itself. The direction in which the force acts, its polarity or sense, is indicated by an arrowhead. This symbol, called a *vector*, is used extensively in electrocardiography to represent forces, both instantaneous and the average of a series (waves). Magnitude is rarely important, sense is indicated by an arrowhead, and the figures at the bottom of the worksheet are used to express direction in three dimensions. Most readers will be familiar with these figures already, and their derivation is discussed in Chapter Five. In their simplest form they should be thought of as three mutually perpendicular lines that define space (Fig. 2-3).

The *projection of a vector* can be compared to its shadow projected on a line (lead) from a light source directed perpendicular to the line (Fig. 2-4). If the vector is perpendicular to the line, it casts no shadow at all; if parallel, the shadow is maximal; the length of the shadow depends on the angle of the vector with the line. In electrocardiography, all forces are treated as rays extending outward from the central point (zero the "B point"), through which all lead lines pass, and the projection of a vector on any lead is determined by dropping a perpendicular from its end to the line of the lead. If it is directed toward the positive pole, it produces an upward deflection; the negative pole, a downward one. In Fig. 2-5A, only horizontal and vertical axes are drawn, and a vector and its projections are shown. If the right end of the horizontal line is labeled east, and the top end of the vertical one north, the vector can be described as directed southeast, or to +45°. In Fig. 2-5B, horizontal and vertical are represented as Leads I and aVF, and the positions of the other frontal leads are shown also. If the vector is defined now as representing the mean QRS in the frontal plane, its "axis," in what lead(s)

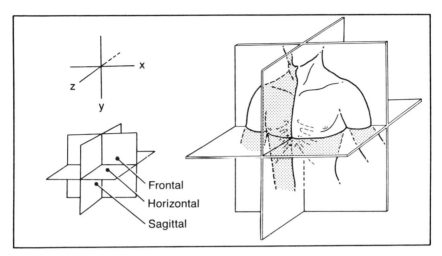

Fig. 2-3. Space is represented by three mutually perpendicular planes.

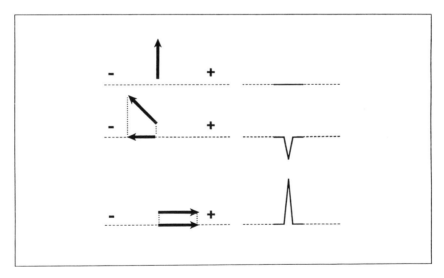

Fig. 2-4. Projection of a vector.

in that tracing would the net QRS area be minimal? In what lead(s) maximal? The tracing is shown in Fig. 2-5C.

One of the most useful things one can do is realize the remarkable validity of Einthoven's premises; they work, leads I and aVF

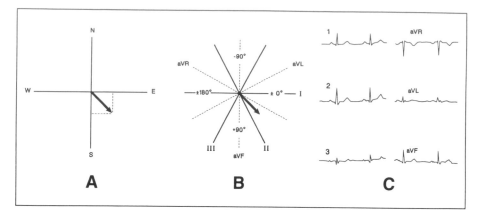

Fig. 2-5. The frontal QRS expressed as a vector.

really are perpendicular to each other, and you can know this from your own experience, not because you saw it in a book. Einthoven did not invent this or cause it to be, but he identified the electrophysiologic features that explain it, and made them available to us (p. 89). It is the way things are, and can be depended on just as water can be depended on to boil at 100°C, apples to fall from trees, and staphylococci to stain blue.

It may help to distinguish between a force as an instantaneous event, and a wave in the tracing as the chart of a progression of forces, and to underscore the significance of the word "mean." Ventricular depolarization is a process, not an event; it occurs over time, some of it in one direction and some in another, and at different rates. To speak of the mean frontal QRS axis treats it as a single value. It has some usefulness, but there is much more information to be had from its components—Q, R, and S. Considering individual waves calls attention to time as a factor, and permits recognition of an abnormality as affecting only the initial part of depolarization, the terminal part, or the whole process, features that may tell the anatomic location of a lesion and are not implicit in axis alone; an axis of +90° does not distinguish between a QR in Lead I and an RS, and the difference may be critical.

Another expression of these same principles is shown in Fig. 2-6. The vector represents a force, e.g., depolarization of a muscle

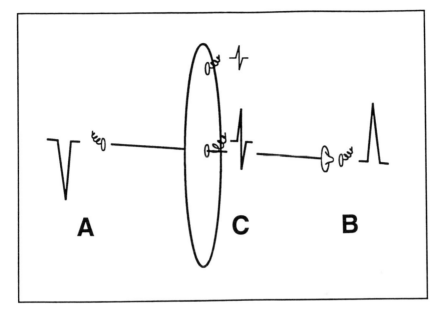

Fig. 2-6. A force approaching the positive pole of a lead writes an upstroke.

strip, recorded from the positive poles of two leads. Observing the convention that a force approaching its positive pole writes an upstroke in that lead, and vice versa, it is easy to see that a positive curve would be recorded in Lead B at the same time that its mirror image is seen in Lead A, the duration of the curves, their width, being a measure of the time it takes the process to go from the left end of the strip to the right. Now consider the curve from a lead whose positive pole is midway between the ends of the vector (C). The first half is upward as the force approaches, and the last half downward as it recedes, a biphasic curve, +/−, with the area subtended by each component equal to that of the other but of opposite sign. This is the transitional curve, transitional, that is, between negative and positive. The vertical line recorded as the process passes directly beneath the electrode is called the "intrinsic" deflection. Amplitude varies inversely with distance, but otherwise the curves recorded from any point on a plane perpendicular to the vector at its midpoint are the same. Now place the midpoint of this vector at the

B point in the center of the system, and consider the transitional plane as infinite in extent. The line defined by its intersection with the surface of the body is called the null pathway, and a curve recorded from any point on it will, of course, be equally biphasic, a transitional, or null, curve.

All this can be summarized: An upstroke in a lead indicates that the positive pole of that lead faces the positive side of a boundary of potential difference. Typically, this means that a force is approaching that pole; a negative deflection, that it is receding from it. An exception is found in some leads when QRS and T are close together in space and T is written as repolarization "backs away" from the positive pole (p. 80). A net area of zero means that the exploring electrode is on a plane perpendicular to the force at its midpoint, and the midpoint is the B point in the center of the chest. This last observation is the key to location of the position of the force in space; it is perpendicular to the line of the lead on which its projection is zero.

One more diagram and admonition. Consider the two curves in Fig. 2-7, A and B. Which represents the larger value? B, of course. The information implicit in a curve is a function of its area, not of either amplitude or duration alone. Most students learn early, however, to estimate the axis from the algebraic sum of the amplitude of R and S in Leads I and III without regard for duration. When the rate of excitation is equal throughout both ventricles, individual waves are so narrow that duration cannot be estimated meaningfully; calculation of area is not a realistic option and can be ignored, but when there is gross discrepancy between the rates of depolarization in different parts of the myocardium, as with right bundle branch block (which does not affect the initial forces but slows and redirects the late ones, *see* p. 159), it becomes critical. When all the limits of all the methods are considered, the axis is inevitably an estimate rather than a precise measure. Computer programs help, but apparently none of them considers area.

5a. QRS orientation: Frontal axis. Now it should be easy to *determine the QRS axis* of the tracing before you. Identify the frontal lead in which the net area of QRS is most nearly zero; that is, the one to which the axis is most nearly perpendicular. If it is aVL, for instance, the direction is either +60° or −120°. Look at the net value

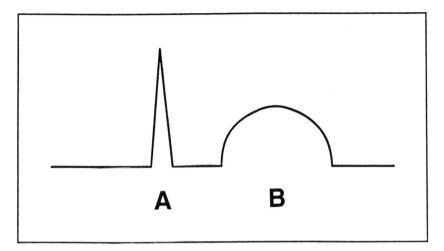

Fig. 2-7. Two values. Which is greater?

of QRS in another lead to tell which. Any will do, because their angular relation to each other is known, but we are accustomed to thinking in terms of orthogonal coordinates, i.e., left–right and up–down, and it is logical to look at I or aVF. If QRS is positive in either, the answer is +60°; negative, –120°. If the area is not clearly smaller in one lead than the others, choose the two in which it is least and take the difference between them as the axis. Say, for instance, the area is clearly smaller in III and aVL than the others but positive in both, and positive in Lead I; the axis is not either +30° or +60°, but +45° would be an reasonable compromise. In the tracing in Fig. 2-8, the frontal QRS axis is about +75°.

Occasionally the choice cannot be narrowed to two leads— almost any would qualify—and in such a tracing it would be inappropriate to enter a number for axis; put a dash in Space 5a and read about the "S1,2,3 syndrome" (p. 227). Computer programs may call attention to this as "axis none" or "axis indeterminate." As an incidental finding, it has no clinical implication.

In most normal adults, the frontal QRS axis lies between –30° and +105°. And note that to call a position for QRS closer than ±15° is to exceed the limits of the method, like calling the pulse rate 81 with the implication that distinction from 80 has clinical value.

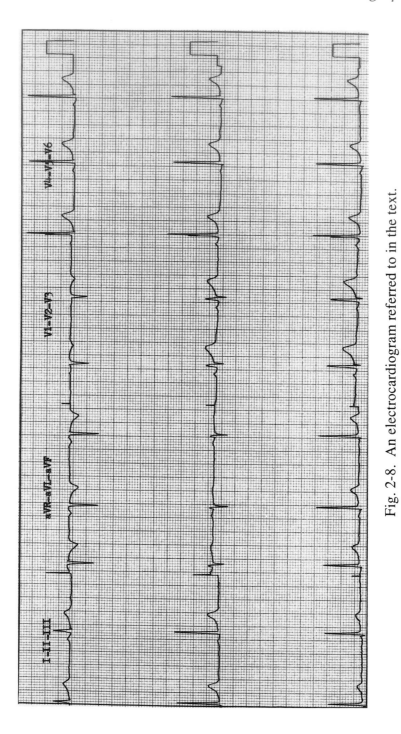

Fig. 2-8. An electrocardiogram referred to in the text.

At this point, the direction of QRS in the *frontal* plane has been determined, but not whether it is directed anteriorly or posteriorly, and this is just as critical as up–down and left–right.

> If the mean frontal QRS is directed to −60° or farther counterclockwise ("left axis deviation"), *see* pp. 162 and 226 for the differential diagnosis; if +105° or farther clockwise ("right axis deviation"), *see* pp. 165 and 226. Orientation of the frontal QRS is a finding and has no clinical implication by itself. It can be compared to describing a patient as lying down or standing up.

5b,c,d. QRS orientation: Horizontal axis. The direction of QRS in the horizontal plane is as important as its direction in the frontal plane and is determined the same way, but with less precision. There is no standard, quantitative reference frame for values in the horizontal plane; the one used on the worksheet is simply a convenient device drawing on the (reasonable) assumptions that V6 (in the midaxillary line) is in the frontal plane, that a line perpendicular to the frontal plane at the B point intersects the surface of the body at the center of the sternum, and that the angle between adjacent precordial leads is 20°. This places the postero-anterior, or Z, lead at V1½, but in clinical reality it is represented well by V1. Efforts to define a truly orthogonal Z lead have not improved upon this arrangement (p. 89). The point in the center of both figures represents the same point in space, zero, the B point. All the lead lines, or axes, pass through it, and all the forces represented in the tracing extend outward from it.

The horizontal axis is assessed by noting the height of R and depth of S in V1 and V6, and identifying the position of the transition from predominantly negative QRSs to predominantly positive ones. Amplitude is given in millimeters (corrected to a standard of 1 mv = 10 mm), e.g., 2:10, 20:2, real values, *not* reduced to the lowest common denominator, *not* 1:5 or 10:1. If there is no R wave, the completely negative character of the complex, a QS, can be indicated by using zero for R and the depth of the complex for S. A normal Q in V6 (p. 41) need not be noted, and an abnormal one will be identified in description of contour. If either lead is missing, a dash can be entered. If figures for a lead other than V1 and V6 are needed, this can be indicated.

In most adults, the complexes are predominantly negative in right precordial leads and positive in those from the left, with an equiphasic one somewhere between; the position of this transition is noted in 5c. Often it is clearly a single lead, typically V4, but just as often it is not. More than one position can be indicated, or a choice can be made by interpolation, e.g., V3-5, V3½.

Now recall the idea of a force expressed as a vector (Fig. 2-6) and note that transition from a negative complex on the right side of the chest, through a biphasic one in the middle, to a positive one on the left is almost exactly like that in the figure. Just as in the frontal plane, the precordial lead in which the QRS area is least, the transitional curve, is the one to which the force is most nearly perpendicular. Say it is V2, as in the tracing in Fig. 2-8. This point on the surface of the chest is on a plane perpendicular to the force at its midpoint (the B point). A line connecting it (the point represented by V2) and the B point in the center of the figure lies in this plane, and a line perpendicular to this one at the B point represents the force, or will when its polarity is indicated by an arrow directed toward the positive curves, usually leftward. All electrical forces generated in the heart are presented by the galvanometer as arising at the B point, and the end of the vector opposite the arrow, its negative side, can be deleted. The magnitude of this vector is rarely of importance; traditionally, it is drawn long; the one for T, to be determined soon, short.

No firm figures can be given for either the limit of the method of this determination or the range of normal. Transition from a negative QRS to a positive one occurs typically at about V4 but may be in any position, and sometimes there is hardly any change at all between V1 and V6 (*see* "S1,2,3," p. 227).

The term "axis" could be used for the postero-anterior direction of QRS as well as the lateral and vertical, but in practice, if attention is called to it at all, it's indicated by the position of the transitional curve, late (more leftward than usual) or early (more rightward), and as broad or abrupt.

QRS orientation: Spatial axis. Now the orientation of QRS in three dimensions is known and, depending on one's ability to draw perspective, it can be indicated roughly in a diagram. Soon the same methods will be used to determine the orientation of T (p. 48); the spatial relation of QRS and T is an important factor in distinguishing normal from abnormal and will be discussed later (p. 51).

5a,b,d. QRS amplitude. The numbers in 5b and 5d, obtained already, serve to document amplitude (voltage) of QRS in the horizontal projection. Voltage is defined as *high* if the sum of the S wave in V1 and the R wave in V5 or V6, whichever is taller, exceeds 3.5 mv, and the limit for determining this figure is about ±5 mm. Voltage is said to be *low* when the amplitude of the *largest* complex in Lead I, II, or III, measured from the highest point above the baseline to the lowest below it, zenith to nadir, is less than 0.5 mv. Note that low voltage is defined in the original "bipolar" leads (p. 86) and can be indicated by writing "low" in space 5a along with orientation.

QRS amplitude can vary considerably from day to day, even from beat to beat, and is influenced by a wide variety of factors other than myocardial mass (p. 228). Voltage, either high or low, is simply a finding, comparable to height, and must be considered in the perspective of all other findings, clinical as well as electrocardiographic, lest a statistical abnormality be given the name of an anatomic or physiologic one. Short stature is not an illness.

The ventricles are depolarized simultaneously, outward from the endocardium (p. 77), and, because left ventricular mass is much greater than right, QRS amplitude is determined largely by the left ventricle. It is tempting to hypothesize a direct relation between muscle mass and voltage, but this is simplistic. *Left ventricular hypertrophy* does sometimes explain high voltage, but voltage is influenced by a host of factors, and there are many, many criteria for high, as well as for hypertrophy, none more "right" than others (p. 192). Sokolow and Lyon's figure for the upper limit of normal, *3.5 mv for the sum of SV1 and RV5 (or RV6, whichever is taller)*

does not exceed 3.5 mv, is probably the most widely used criterion, but whatever EKG measure is proposed is useful only
to the extent that it correlates with anatomic reality, and the
wide diversity of standards for objective, quantitative criteria
for hypertrophy limits the value of all of them. The traditional
definition is increase in cell size, but not many EKG studies
have used this. Some have used wall thickness, as determined
by various means, and others have accepted simply a clinical
diagnosis of a lesion that would overload the left ventricle
selectively. The effect of dilatation is rarely even mentioned.
There is no clean point at which normality ceases and hypertrophy begins, either structurally or in the tracing, and, whatever figures are used, values for normal and abnormal overlap
very widely. The important risk to the patient is that more
significance will be attached to the EKG interpretation than is
justified; restraint is called for. Left ventricular hypertrophy
is a response to disease, not a disease itself, a mechanism for
sustaining cardiac output when a greater than normal load is
imposed by increase of flow and/or resistance. The lesions
that can produce this are recognizable easily on physical examination (p. 196) and are known already by the doctor who has
taken the blood pressure and done a physical examination.
Failing to call left ventricular hypertrophy in the EKG will
not hurt the patient, but calling it when it is not present introduces the risk for at least unhappiness. If perceived as an abnormality itself, instead of as compensation for an abnormality
already known, not recognized as someone's estimate of the
length of a line, it can lead to real problems.

   Criteria for hypertrophy of the *right ventricle* are even
harder to define than those for the left, and affect mostly orientation of QRS; classically, it is directed more ventrad, a tall
R in V1 and deep S in V6. A ventricle may be dilated as well
as hypertrophied, and which change is reflected in the EKG is
not always clear; *enlarged* is often the preferable word (p. 187).
One of the risks associated with the expression *axis deviation*
is that right axis deviation may be assumed to represent right
ventricular hypertrophy, and left equated with left ventricular
hypertrophy. This is not justified, and is even more inappro-

priate when applied to the right ventricle than to the left, especially when it is realized that the right ventricle is more anterior than right (p. 193).

Low voltage, too, is a finding that has no clinical importance by itself but may be an important part of the picture when all factors are considered. It often seems to be assumed that it means pericardial effusion, and this is, indeed, to be considered, but there are many other possible explanations, and "low" means different things to different people, especially in the precordial leads where no widely used figures can be cited (p. 228). There are instances, such as evaluating the effects of some drugs used in treating malignant neoplasia, and detecting rejection of cardiac transplants, when diminution of voltage from control values is a useful observation, but this calls for special techniques and is not relevant to interpretation of routine tracings.

5e. QRS contour. An adjective commonly entered for contour is "wide," but this describes duration, not shape, and duration has been noted quantitatively already in 2a. Contour means configuration, form, what it looks like. It is a statement of the continually changing direction and amplitude of a series of instantaneous vectors, and the rate at which these changes occur, and can be described only by adjectives. The *normal* QRS may consist of only one curve, a QS or an R, or include three or more, depending on the lead. There is no conspicuous difference in the duration of waves of comparable magnitude in normals, and they are all composed of straight lines and sharp angles, i.e., clean. In a lead in which it is mostly unidirectional, usually aVL, I, II, V6, aVF, and/or III, the prototype QRS consists of a tall R, often followed by a small S and sometimes initiated by a narrow (less than 0.03 s), sharply defined Q whose depth is usually less than about 10% of the amplitude of R but may be more (p. 77). If these qualities are present, and those described below are absent, the adjective for space 5e is "normal."

Abnormality of contour may be limited to the first part of the complex, the last, or it may be diffuse. *Initial abnormality* can be described as a slur, for instance, i.e, slowing of the rate of deflection with widening of the trace, or a notch, i.e., abrupt, sharp change in direction, e.g., a wide, notched, or slurred, Q in a specified lead (in another lead it would be an R). Abnormality of the *terminal part selectively* often affects contour and orientation, as well as duration, and presents as a broad, slurred wave directed to the right (S1) and anteriorly (terminal RV1) (p. 159), or is limited to counterclockwise direction with little if any change in duration or contour (p. 162). The complex may be wide and slurred throughout (p. 160), or there may be small notches in any part of it *(see below)*. Duration of QRS as a whole has been noted (2d), but that of its components has to be covered by description of individual waves; a wide Q has a different meaning from a wide R or S, and knowledge that the complex as a whole is wide does not tell which part of it is abnormal.

Both *smooth* and *clean* as characteristics of the normal QRS are relative, and the range of normal is wide. Some lesions, typically myocardial infarction (p. 174) and ventricular pre-excitation (p. 155), are expressed in the initial phase selectively, for instance, while others, such as right bundle branch block (p. 159) and left anterior fascicular block (p. 162), deform only the terminal forces; left bundle branch block often affects the whole complex (p. 160). Widening associated with drugs and electrolytes (pp. 230, 231) is diffuse, producing no localized change of contour. Unusual examples of abnormalities limited to late forces include the prominent "J" or "Osborn" wave of hypothermia (p. 237), and "late potentials" (p. 184). Notches, like spots on the skin, are common. A notch no more makes an abnormality than a râle makes pneumonia or a robin a spring; some notching can be found in any tracing, and is seen especially in transitional leads, typically Lead III and a midprecordial lead. What is outside the limits of normal is a learned judgment.

Function

Abnormality of function, of physiology, may produce change in the more sensitive parts of the tracing, representing repolarization, although not being apparent in the more stable parts written by depolarization.

Atria

Atrial repolarization has been invoked as explanation for part of the pattern of flutter (p. 130), and sometimes one sees reference to a P_t, or a T_a, but it is not generally identifiable in the surface tracing. Atrial infarcts occur and must produce change in P and the PQ segment (p. 185).

Ventricles

The T wave, or ST-T complex, a continuous line written by repolarization of the ventricles, is divided arbitrarily into an initial portion, ST, and a terminal one, T. There is not a point at which ST ends and T begins, but it is possible to separate them to a useful degree for descriptive purposes, much as day (sun-up to sun-down) is separated from night (sun-down to sun-up). *Day* also refers to a period of 24 hours, and in everyday conversation it is easy to tell which is meant. Similarly, *T* may refer to the whole curve or to the distal part selectively: ST-T leaves no doubt.

The importance of describing the ST-T complex carefully lies in the specificity–sensitivity spectrum of the ventricular tracing. This can be compared to a pennant on a pole (Fig. 2-9), in which the pole represents QRS and the tip of the pennant T. Any little breeze that comes along can move the tip of the pennant, but it takes a much stronger wind to straighten out the proximal part, and a real hurricane to bend the pole. In either case, the pennant will return to its original dependent position when the wind subsides. In the first two instances, its original (normal) relation to the pole will have been restored also; in the last, the pennant is intrinsically normal but its relation to the pole is not, a secondary abnormality, the primary abnormality is in the pole, not the pennant (pp. 48, 80, 201). The T wave is the most sensitive and least specific part of the repolarization complex, and abnormality limited to it is nonspecific. ST is less sensitive; abnormal displacement here translates almost quantitatively to myocardial injury, but is still less than specific. Abnormality of QRS almost always means anatomic abnormality in the ventricular wall, and ST-T abnormality may reflect this rather than intrinsic functional change.

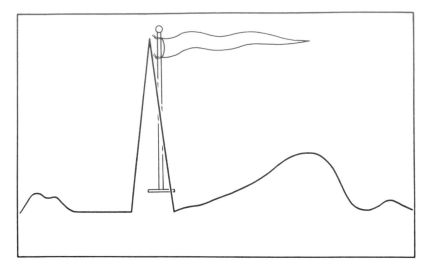

Fig. 2-9. The sensitivity–specificity spectrum of QRS-T-U is like a pennant on a pole.

Description of the ST segment can be compared to description of an egg on a table; two things must be handled, the position of something in space and its shape. In both cases, position can be defined quantitatively and easily by the distance in each of three dimensions from a fixed reference point, but shape is subjective and requires adjectives. The egg is round, elliptical, or somewhere in between, depending on the view, but what we are talking about is an egg, and, because everybody knows what an egg looks like, it is enough to describe it as *egg-shaped*. A comparable compromise would be to describe the normal ST contour as simply that, normal, and indeed this is what is done most of the time, but in this case the meaning of *normal* does not draw on quite the same universal understanding that *egg-shaped* does, and to define it as the absence of abnormal does not help much. The following paragraphs propose solutions.

Line 6

6a. ST Displacement and contour. The position of ST in space, its *orientation*, is defined by the position of a point, J, relative to the fixed point at the center of the system, the B point (represented in a series of beats by the baseline, p. 9); it is at the baseline, above it, or below it. *Amplitude* is indicated by how far above or below. In most normals it is at, or very near, the baseline, and departure from this is indicated as slight, moderate, or marked. *Duration* is included with that of T as the QT interval.

Whether elevation or depression is outside the limits of normal is determined by the ratio of its amplitude to the that of QRS and T, change from previous tracings, and, especially, the *contour of the line that follows J*, variables cannot be quantified very precisely. Some ST elevation, especially when its contour is normal and T is tall, is common in both right and left precordial leads in normals. It usually elicits no comment when seen in V1-2-3 but is called *early repolarization* when seen in V4-5-6 (p. 205).

6b. ST Contour. Description of contour is a little more difficult, and another analogy to physical examination may help. When medical students first write up physical examinations, it is not enough to describe the skin as simply normal. In those first few efforts, a long litany of things that are absent is expected, e.g., macules, papules, excoriations, spider angiomata, and silvery imbricated scales, as well as a description of turgor, color, temperature, and other characteristics. This is in order to fix in the students' minds features of the skin that they had not known about, or at least had not been in the habit of thinking about, until then. Soon, though, it becomes acceptable to describe the skin as normal. Description of ST is similar. What is being described is a line in space, and it looks different from different views. It is almost necessary to fall back on *normal* if no abnormality is present, but to do this requires understanding, not only of what is normal, but also of what forms abnormality may take. This is one of the areas in which lack of standard EKG terminology is most noticeable, especially the common failure to distinguish between displacement and contour, the position of a point and the shape of a line.

One way to describe the normal ST-T contour is this. By the time the QRS has been written, repolarization has begun, but very little voltage has been generated, and the trace is still at, or very near, the baseline in most leads. It then departs from that level at an increasingly rapid rate, becomes T somewhere along the way, reaches a maximum amplitude, and returns quickly to the baseline. Note that this description does not take sign (orientation) into account; the same process may produce a negative curve in aVR, for instance, a positive one in aVF, and not be identifiable at all in aVL (Fig. 2-8), or, with a slightly different orientation, negative in aVR, flat in V1, and positive in V6. The proximal part of this line, the ST segment, is principally horizontal, and abnormality in it is described by adjectives that relate to that characteristic; the distal part, T, by adjectives that relate to verticality.

In practice, description of contour is inherently subjective and imprecise. The difficulty is illustrated by some of the expressions in use: J depression, cove-planing, ischemic, upsloping, and downsloping. *J depression* fails to recognize that there are two features to be described, displacement and contour. The position of J is what defines depression/elevation (orientation and amplitude); J depression is the only kind of depression there is. The probable implication is that there is no abnormality of contour, and that the displacement is of little consequence. *Cove-planing* is an attempt to recognize the second feature, the shape of the line that follows J, but has little meaning (as defined by something that can be looked up in a dictionary). *Planar*, used sometimes, is better to the extent that it suggests flatness, but *ischemic* invokes an explanation for a finding without saying what the finding is. *Upsloping* apparently has the same connotation as *normal*, and *downsloping* is included in the definition of flat but is less quantitative.

Abnormality of contour can be indicated pretty well in most cases as sagging, arched, flat, or straightened (Fig. 2-10), either generally or in specified leads (p. 206). If T voltage is so low that there is virtually no T, ST is flat by default, but the abnormality is in T, the distal end of the process, the most sensitive and least specific part, not ST, and this can be indicated by describing the ST contour (space 6b) as "related to T" or "see below," referring to Line Seven, where an abnormality will be described. If ST is flat in the presence of normal T voltage, it can be described as just that, flat.

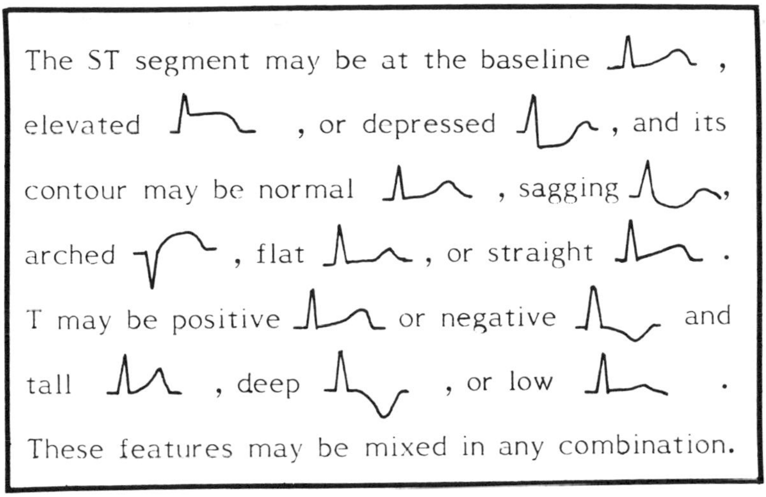

The ST segment may be at the baseline ⏜, elevated ⏜, or depressed ⏜, and its contour may be normal ⏜, sagging ⏜, arched ⏜, flat ⏜, or straight ⏜. T may be positive ⏜ or negative ⏜ and tall ⏜, deep ⏜, or low ⏜. These features may be mixed in any combination.

Fig. 2-10. ST-T contours. *See also* Fig. 13-3.

When ST displacement is abnormal, it translates directly to the everyday word *injury* with its clear meaning of impairment of function, in this case electrophysiologic function, without any implication of etiology. *Injury* is a word from the common language that retains its meaning here. A newspaper report of "damage in the millions, but no injuries" assumes that the reader will understand *damage* to refer to inanimate objects, and *injury* to living ones; specifically, people. It will be understood, also, that *injury* implies impairment of function, not cessation of it, and that injury is transient; injured tissue either recovers or dies. A lesion of function is to be distinguished from one of structure, as sprain is from fracture, angina from infarct. Myocardial injury can be identified often as deep or superficial (p. 202), and, when the clinical setting is known, this can be very helpful; processes that injure the superficial layers of the myocardium without involving the deep ones are usually different from those that injure deep layers while sparing superficial ones. An important pattern to be considered in the differential of ST displacement is *early repolarization* (p. 205), which is normal.

Line 7

The ST-T complex is a continuous curve, and the farther to the right one goes the harder it becomes to describe it precisely; orientation, duration, amplitude, and contour are still the characteristics to be assessed, but the criteria by which they are judged, and the words used to describe them, become increasingly vague.

7a. T orientation (axis): Frontal. Orientation of T is determined exactly as that for QRS or any other wave or deflection. Find the frontal lead in which the net area subtended by T is least. If one is not clearly different from the others, indicate this by a dash in 7a; if T voltage is just too low to justify description, write "low," not only telling that the T axis cannot be calculated but also explaining why, and naming an abnormality. In the tracing in Fig. 2-8, T is smallest in Lead aVL, meaning that it is perpendicular to that lead. It is headed toward either +60° or –120°. Now note its sign (projection) in Lead I or aVF. If it is positive in either, the answer is +60°; negative, –120°. Clearly, the answer is +60°, but this does not mean it could not have been called could be +45° or +75° just as easily.

No firm figure can be given for the limit of the method for orientation of T, but certainly it cannot be called any closer than ±15°.

> Whether orientation of T is normal or abnormal depends on its spatial relation to QRS, and the horizontal projection is just as important as the frontal (Line Nine).

7b. T orientation (axis): Horizontal. The direction of T in the horizontal plane is determined the same way as that of any component of the tracing, by locating the transitional curve; but documentation is a little different. Unlike the QRS, in which three names, Q, R, and S, are available for naming only two directions, up and down, T is always called just T, whether it is positive, negative, or biphasic, and it is easy to choose one of these for each position. Fill in the blanks in 7b with +, ⊖, or ±, demonstrating the position of the transition curve, or that there is not one. One of the few things in the electrocardiogram that change with age is orientation of QRS and

T. At birth, the QRS is directed clockwise and anteriorly, and with age it moves counterclockwise and posteriorly. T follows the opposite course and is likely to be positive in all precordial leads by adulthood or before. T voltage may be so low in all leads that to call it either positive or negative would be specious, and this can be described by entering ± in the blank for each lead, documenting an abnormality that will be named in the interpretation on Line Thirteen.

When a transition curve for T can be located (by interpolation if necessary; extrapolation is more risky), it identifies a point on the chest that is on a plane perpendicular to the unknown force and equidistant from its ends. In the tracing in Fig. 2-8, it is between V1 and V2, say V1$^1/_2$. A line through this point and the B point is perpendicular to the force. Draw this line, extending it beyond the boundaries of the circle to emphasize that it represents the intersection of two planes, not the force; it is not a vector. Next, construct a perpendicular to it at B. This is the T vector. (As with the QRS, amplitude is not usually considered; T is drawn short and QRS long). All that remains to complete the figure is to put a point on one end to indicate the direction in which repolarization occurs, i.e., toward the leads with positive T. Whether this is normal depends on its relation to QRS, the QRS-T angle, or ventricular gradient, and will be discussed later (Line Nine). All cardiac vectors arise at the B point, and the negative side of this line can be deleted.

T orientation (axis): Spatial. Now the direction of the mean T in all three dimensions has been determined, and is shown in the two figures at the bottom of the worksheet. As with the QRS (p. 39), an attempt should be made to show the spatial orientation in a single figure.

Normality or abnormality of T is a function of both its intrinsic characteristics (amplitude and contour) and its spatial relation to QRS, and often the latter can be represented only roughly. The direction of T in the horizontal plane is only an approximation at best, because of the absence of a standard scale in degrees, and because very often, especially in adults, T is positive in all precordial leads. The patterns in leads aVR and V6 are often nearly equal and opposite, though, representing views of the process from opposite ends (Fig. 2-6), and a flat T in V1 can be seen as transitional when TaVR is negative and T V6 is positive.

Duration of T is included in QT.

Amplitude and Contour of T. T voltage (amplitude) is described as normal, low, or high. A good criterion for *low* is that it is less than about 10% of QRS in a lead in which QRS is completely positive or negative and T is of the same sign. When it is low in frontal leads, this can be noted in space 7a along with, or instead of, the figure for orientation in degrees, and in precordial leads by ± or as "low," in addition to the sign, in each lead. When voltage is *high*, T is described as "tall," or "deep," in appropriate leads. There is no really good definition for high voltage, how tall or how deep the wave must be to merit that description, but 50% of the amplitude of QRS in a lead in which both are of the same sign is a good figure from which to start. *Contour* may be described as rounded when voltage is low, but usually is not mentioned at all. Symmetry is the most important abnormality of contour, but when T is tall this may be more apparent than real, because the difference between the rate at which the trace departs from the baseline, and that at which it returns to it, is not so easy to see as when T voltage is normal. Remember, ST and T are parts of the same curve, and another way to make T symmetrical is to flatten ST. Both factors may be at work.

No ST-T pattern is specific, more than one interpretation is possible for all of them, but there are two common ones that are expressed predominantly in T and, by themselves, are at least suggestive of explanations. (1) When duration, amplitude, and contour are normal, but T is negative in leads with positive QRSs, and positive in those with negative QRSs, it is likely that the left ventricle is overloaded. (2) When the contour of T is symmetrical, especially if its orientation is dorsad; i.e., there is a negative, symmetrical T in midprecordial leads, coronary insufficiency is the probable explanation. These two patterns are not mutually exclusive. *See* p. 212.

Line 8

The U wave. Amplitude and orientation of U are indicated as with other waves, but its contour is always pretty much the same, and its duration cannot be estimated usefully—just a small, slow wave. When it calls for comment at all, "prominent" will usually suffice. It may be merged with T and read as a long QT interval. This should be suspected whenever QT is called much longer than 0.44 s, no matter what the rate, and often can be confirmed by finding a "dimple" where the curves merge, usually seen best in a right precordial lead. The only time orientation of U is noted is when it is negative in midprecordial leads.

Abnormality of U is not rare, but is even less specific, and harder to define, than T abnormality. Negativity in midprecordial leads is often associated with negativity of T in the same leads, suggesting coronary insufficiency (p. 217), and prominence is often found with hypokalemia (p. 231). It is suspected that U may be related to delayed after-depolarizations (p. 235), as well as to repolarization, and that abnormality here may explain ventricular ectopy in some cases (p. 184).

Other

Line 9

Spatial QRS-T angle (ventricular gradient). The potential relevance to the patient of every characteristic of the tracing, normal and abnormal, must be considered, not only by itself but also in the context provided by all others, change from previous tracings, and the clinical picture as a whole. Everything is related to everything else, and change in one component may affect the meaning of others. Clearly, it is no more possible to list all potential interrelations and interpretations here than it is for the results of the history and physical examination, but the objective of the present exercise is to demonstrate how to identify the problem and, that having been done, to point the way to interpretation of it in a clinically useful fashion.

The first step is to establish the spatial relation between QRS and T, the *ventricular gradient*, or $\hat{G}$ (p. 80), a useful combination of two variables comparable to habitus on physical examination. Think of a man seven feet tall. Wouldn't everybody agree that he is tall? How about one who weighs 200 pounds? Would there be equal agreement that he is fat? Not necessarily. It depends on how tall he is, how old he is, what kind of condition he is in, and perhaps other factors. The spatial relation of QRS and T is inescapably considered in evaluating a tracing, just as habitus is on physical examination, but, also like habitus, it is not always identified in the record. The QRS, like height, can be compared to a template drawn from experience without reference to its T, but T cannot be evaluated without taking the QRS pattern into account. Many factors are involved in determining the order of repolarization of the ventricular myocardium, but one that must always be considered is the order of depolarization; if its course is altered, that of repolarization must be, too.

Primary ST-T abnormality, evidence of change in myocardial function not manifest in QRS, is chiefly in the intrinsic characteristics of the curve, duration, amplitude, and contour; secondary, mostly orientation (p. 201). It is possible, of course, for there to be both primary and secondary abnormality, but, because none of these features is specific, it is difficult to know when such an interpretation is justified (*see* p. 160).

9a. Frontal. The angle between QRS and T in the frontal plane is implicit in the figures recorded in spaces 5a and 7a. If, for instance, QRS is at +30° and T is at +60°, the angle between them is 30°; if +30° and −15°, 45°. (Note that orientation of QRS and T designates the direction of rays emanating from the center of a circle, and requires a plus or a minus sign, but that the size of the angle is a value and does not have a sign.)

9b. Horizontal. Estimation of the horizontal QRS-T angle is based on the assumption of a 20° angle between contiguous leads, a useful device but one with no very scientific base (p. 89). Look at the vectors you have constructed to represent QRS and T in the figure for the horizontal plane at the bottom of the worksheet. Each is perpendicular to its null plane, of course, and those planes were determined by location of the transitional curve on the chest. Assume that the QRS transition is at about V2, T transition at V1^1/$_2$, and both forces are directed to the left. The horizontal QRS-T angle is approx 10° (Fig. 2-8). If QRS had been positive in V6 and negative in V1, and T positive in V1 and negative in V6, it would have been 170°.

In normals, QRS and T are close together in space, not more than about 45° apart in the frontal plane and 60° in the horizontal. Recognizing ±15° as the limit of the method for locating QRS, and that the figure for T is even less accurate, it is easy to expand this to 65°, and even much beyond that, depending on stability of the findings, clinical setting, and judgment, but it is important to be aware that choices are being made so that they can be made responsibly.

The orientation of both QRS and T in each of three dimensions will have been indicated in the two diagrams at the bottom of the worksheet. If they are combined in a single figure, with the arrowheads drawn to show perspective, the concept of spatial relation of depolarization and repolarization will be clear, and it will become even more meaningful as similar figures are constructed for tracings with different abnormalities. The ventricular gradient is always a factor as interpretation evolves, but is not often named.

Other combinations to be considered in interpretation. Some examples of the interpretive process are listed below. Clinical decision making is not something that can be described step by step in a strictly linear order beginning here and ending there, but requires cognitive procedures that have been described as like "tangled webs."[9,14] It cannot be computerized fully, and it is important to be aware that interpretation of an electrocardiogram is an example of this. On the bottom line, electrocardiography is no more absolute than any other clinical discipline; it is up to the doctor to do the right thing.

Before a definitive conclusion is reached, the present findings must be compared to those in previous tracings, just as the old chart must be reviewed in order for present complaints can be evaluated in context, but, in the interests of objectivity, a tentative interpretation of the new one by itself should be reached first. When previous ones have been reviewed, this may have to be changed, but prior knowledge of how they were interpreted can interfere with objectivity in describing the new one.

Abnormality of QRS translates directly to anatomic abnormality in the ventricular wall in most cases, or the anatomic locus of a functional one. If it is prolonged *and* a certain contour is present *and* the mechanism is sinus and uncomplicated, there is right bundle branch block, *but* if the mechanism is sinus at rate 85 and the QRS rate is 30 with regular rhythm, there is complete AV block and the pattern locates the default pacemaker in the left ventricle. If the ventricular rate is 200, the same pattern may be evidence of either left ventricular origin, or of right bundle branch block in addition to usurping atrial ectopy. Findings may be innocuous in themselves but part of a bigger picture that is not; ventricular rate 80 with regular rhythm and a narrow QRS sounds like a sinus mechanism, but if the atrial rate is 320 the significance is very different. (What if the atrial rate is 90?)

Low T voltage is an abnormality by itself, and so is direction of the frontal QRS to –60°, but that is all that can be said for sure about either observation alone. Like fever and leukocytosis, they are only findings, but findings can be assembled in groups to produce a whole that is more than the sum of its parts. A certain distortion of the initial part of QRS is typical of a scar deep in the myocardium, for instance, and a certain combination of ST-T abnormalities is typical of myocardial injury. To submit these as separate interpretations, #1 deep scar and #2 myocardial injury, would be accurate but not very useful; to combine them as evidence of an acute infarct, which may also explain abnormality of QRS orientation if present (left anterior fascicular block), and low T voltage, would be more useful but requires three assumptions: that the most likely explanation for a scar in that position is indeed the proper one in this case, that the same lesion explains the injury, and that

injury is transient. That is combining two potentially unrelated findings and attributing etiology, going far beyond what
is known from the tracing alone, playing statistics, practicing
medicine. If the patient is a 70-year-old man who had an infarct
five years ago, the interpretation might be changed to an old
infarct with a ventricular aneurysm (pp. 180, 185); if he is 20
years old with no complaints, the whole picture may reflect
idiopathic hypertrophic subaortic stenosis, the scar of a ventricular myomectomy, or something else.

An S1,2,3 pattern (p. 227) may be normal or evidence of
right ventricular enlargement, a myocardial infarct, or something else. More than one interpretation of almost any finding
is possible, and the significance of one that is equivocal by
itself may be clear when seen as part of a bigger picture. If
there is evidence of right atrial enlargement, for instance, the
S1,2,3 pattern probably represents right ventricular enlargement, and, if the patient is a 60-year-old man with pulmonary
emphysema and pneumonia, the likelihood is even greater—
but the pattern, the finding, has not changed.

If an abnormality has been identified and its meaning is not
clear, name it. To name a problem gives one a measure of control over it; the answer can be looked up. Try the index. Ask for
help. In making a diagnosis, all the information available must
be taken into account, and one of the limiting factors in the practice of electrocardiography is that interpreters rarely know all
they need in order to be as helpful as they might be. Remember
the definition of the practice of medicine (p. 5); it can be para-
phrased as doing the right thing even when the information
needed to decide what that is is not available. Whether there is
input from the primary doctor or not, the secondary one is still
bound by the first rule, do nothing that would hurt the patient.

Line 10

Comparison to previous tracings. After a tentative interpretation has been reached, in clinical context to the extent that is known,
but being careful not to assume too much, the tracing must be compared to previous ones, and the words used in the reports of those

are important factors. There is often information in differences between tracings not inherent in a single one, and it is almost always possible to say the same thing in different words, as well as to interpret the same data in a different way. Without awareness of what has been said before, there is risk of introducing an unnecessary element of consternation in the mind of the doctor who reads the report and acts on it. Words can hurt and must be handled carefully. Never, never forget to consider technical error.

The interpretation can be modified as often as necessary to incorporate new information, but somewhere along the line a conclusion must be reached, a statement of what the tracing says about three subjects: (1) the anatomy and (2) the physiology of atria and ventricles, and (3) the interplay of events in these two electrical systems, the mechanism.

This statement may be brief or complicated but must be worded so that the doctor to whom it is addressed can relate it to signs or symptoms. It should be supplemented with any brief comment that will make it more helpful.

Interpretation

Line 11

Mechanism. One of the few things that is absolutely consistent in the traditional reporting of EKGs is that the "rhythm," i.e., the mechanism, is named first, identifying the focus driving the atria, that driving the ventricles, the rate and rhythm of each, and the causal relationship between them, or its absence. It may require several statements: (1) sinus mechanism, rate 80; (2) third degree AV block; (3) PVCs; (4) artificial ventricular pacemaker firing and capturing appropriately, rate 70, or (5) it may be covered completely with "(1) sinus mechanism, rate 80."

An explanation for a named abnormality of mechanism is relevant, and is to be considered, but is a separate step that, theoretically, should be included as a supplementary comment. In practice, however, this distinction is not always respected, especially when there is supraventricular ectopy.

Line 12

Structure. Structure is handled second. Information in P and QRS represents anatomic features of atria and ventricles, and if there is no abnormality of orientation, duration, amplitude, or contour of either, there is no reason to suspect structural abnormality of these chambers. A statement to this effect would be logical, but in practice is not required or expected, and the report can proceed without comment about structure.

Line 13

Function. The ST-T-U is dealt with last. This is the part of the tracing that represents function, physiology, the most sensitive and least specific part. If there is no abnormality here, and none in either the mechanism, P, or QRS, the second and third components of the report can be combined in a single statement that the tracing is within normal limits; if an abnormality of mechanism has been noted, *otherwise* within normal limits.* If ST-T abnormality is interpreted as secondary to QRS abnormality, the third component may be omitted with the assumption that it has been covered already, or "otherwise within normal limits" can be added.

All ST-T abnormalities are nonspecific, but they often fall into useful patterns. Observing the rule to be as specific as possible, and know how specific that is, it is customary to say that there are ST-T abnormalities (fact) and follow this with whatever speculation or suggestion is appropriate, e.g., suggestive of a given explanation, enough to make it probable, or simply nonspecific. Examples:

1. ST-T abnormalities, suggestive of coronary insufficiency.
2. ST-T abnormalities, probably evidence of left ventricular overload.
3. ST-T abnormalities, probably evidence of coronary insufficiency and/or left ventricular overload.
4. ST-T abnormalities, nonspecific.

Otherwise in this context follows statement of mechanism. It can be seen as implying that the mechanism is abnormal, but is intended instead to cover both of the *other* components of the interpretation, structure and function, with one statement; mechanism is always identified first whether it is abnormal or not.

Reservations such as "possible," "consistent with," "cannot rule out," "compatible with," "appears to be," and similar expressions that introduce possibilities without naming alternatives, must not be used. What is known in each category should be made clear and supplemented by comments deemed to be helpful to the primary doctor in putting the information in clinical context. Three levels of confidence are recognized: suggestive, probable, and confident (i.e., virtually certain, actionable). "Typical" and "characteristic" are in a different category; flattened depression of precordial ST is typical of coronary insufficiency, for instance, but the clinical setting and stability of the finding must be taken into account in application of that fact. The limiting factor in the precision with which the interpretation can be stated is the need to express all these things in idiomatic doctor-talk.

When the answer is simply not clear, as is often the case, to be as specific as possible may call for bracketing: "(1) Probably within normal limits, at worst only small ST-T abnormalities," or "(1) Nonspecific ST-T abnormalities, (2) Suggests old anterior myocardial infarct." In each case the statement respects the limits of the method. "Probably within normal limits" is an incomplete statement that will not stand alone; the alternative must be specified. If the diagnosis of old anterior infarct can be made with confidence, it is not necessary to make a separate diagnosis of ST-T abnormality in most cases. It is the same logic that prevails in any other diagnosis, e.g., "Fever of undetermined origin, suspect brucellosis." If the diagnosis of brucellosis were firm, it would not be necessary to mention fever separately; when the diagnosis is secure, its components are implicit.

Jargon that fails to meet the criteria for relevance to the patient, even though widely used, is not acceptable as an interpretation, e.g., "left (or right) axis deviation," "early repolarization," "poor progression of the R wave."

After the full worksheet has been completed for a few tracings, it can be abbreviated to the no-frills form, derived in Fig. 2-11 and demonstrated in Fig. 2-12, suitable for notation on the tracing itself, just as the long form for physical examination with which beginning students contend is shortened with experience. In the short form, there are no labels and no decimal points; the spacing of information identifies it.

EKG WORKSHEET

Patient Information

(1) Name   ID Number   Date and time tracing made

     a   DOE, Jane   b   123,456   c   month - day - year

Mechanism

(2) Rates/minute and intervals in hundredths of a second.

     Atria: a __65__   Vents: b __65__   PR: c __16__   QRS: d __08__   QT: e __40__

(3) Pacemaker   AV   Pacemaker   supra-
     for atria: a __sinus__   conduction: b __1:1__   for ventricles: c __ventricular__

Structure

(4) Atria
     (P): __directed left and caudad__

(5) Vents (QRS):   frontal   RV1:SV1   Transition   RV6:SV6   Contour

     a+25 °   b _3_ : _15_   c _3½_   d 25 : 0   e __normal__

Function

(6) ST: Displacement (the position of a point, J) a __none__

     Contour (the shape of a line) b __normal__

(7) T: Frontal a +60 °,   Precordial b __neg__ V1, __+__ V2, __+__ V3, __+__ V4, __+__ V5, __+__ V6

(8) U: not remarkable (x), other __--__

Other

(9) QRS-T angle: Frontal a __15__ °,   Horizontal b __40__ °

(10) Change since tracing of date/time: __--__ , __--__

Interpretation

(11) Mechanism: __Sinus, rate 65__

(12) Structure: __Within normal limits__

(13) Function: __Within normal limits__

All leads are labeled
at their positive poles

A

Interpreted by: _____ Signature _____   Date: month - day - year

Fig. 2-11. An applied summary of Chapter Two *(continued on following page).*

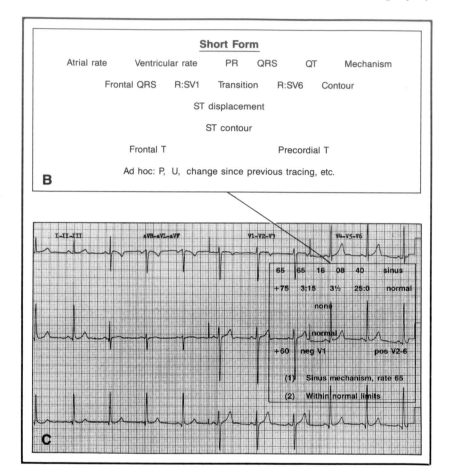

Fig. 2-11. *(continued)*.

Now you have completed the "physical diagnosis" part of electrocardiography and are ready to use it in evaluation of tracings
from your patients, referring to the other parts of this book, and all
other books, for help with the problems you identify, just as you
would use textbooks of medicine and surgery. The first and most
critical objective is to name the problem; if you can do that, you can
probably look up the answer. The index will lead you to the discussion in the book, and the text there will lead you to the literature.

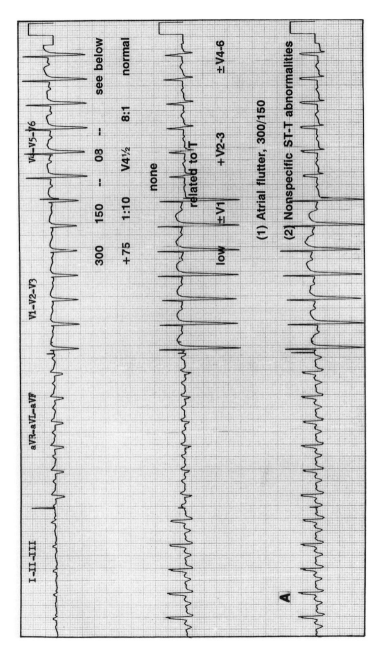

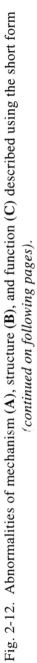

Fig. 2-12. Abnormalities of mechanism (**A**), structure (**B**), and function (**C**) described using the short form *(continued on following pages)*.

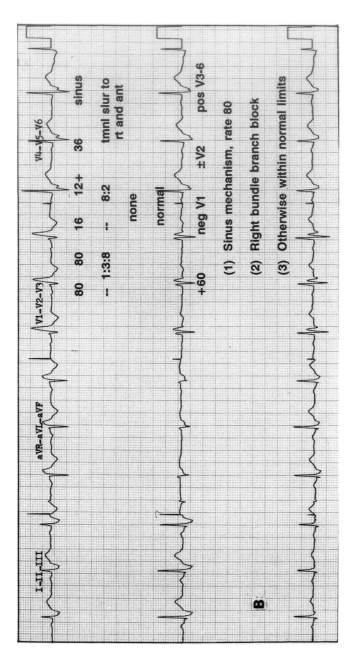

Fig. 2-12. (continued).

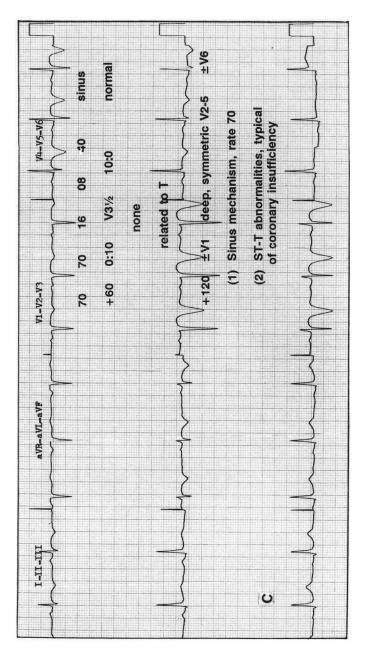

Fig. 2-12. (*continued*).

THREE

Electrocardiography in Perspective

This chapter is designed to place electrocardiography in clinical and historic perspective by reviewing its development in the reference frame of clinical medicine of the past one hundred years.

An electrocardiogram, a record of the electrical activity of the heart, is a graph of voltage against time, and correlation of its elements with information from history, physical examination, X-ray, autopsy, and other studies has given it very great clinical value. It is produced by a machine that "reads the secrets of the heart"[23, 700] and writes them out for all to see, using an 8-letter alphabet (P, Q, R, S, T, U, and sometimes B and J), less flexible than the 26-letter one of English, but effective and translatable into other languages. ECG is a reasonable and acceptable abbreviation of the English *electrocardiogram*, as well as of its Latin roots, but the original word was German, *Elektrokardiogramm*, and EKG is the traditional abbreviation; Einthoven wrote it E. K. G.

Electrocardiography is a medical specialty in which one doctor interprets a laboratory study for another, similar in many respects to Pathology and Radiology. A pathologist looking at a tissue section through a microscope, though, examines something obviously real, a part of the patient, and a radiologist studying a chest film looks at a picture of a part of the patient, but an electrocardiographer works with a symbol of a concept. Electricity generated in the heart is just as real as tissue and pictures, but more abstract. Any information it contains must be converted to words to have meaning, and the nomenclature used for this is so well known that it may take conscious effort to realize that a symbol is not the thing symbolized;[571] there are no Q waves in the heart. Despite this, electrocardiography ranks with history, physical examination, and X-ray as a fundamental method of examination of the heart. Its immediate value is small in most cases, just as the immediate value of most white counts is small, and most visits to the doctor for that matter, but, also as with these, it may be critical. Almost everyone has an electrocardiogram at some time, and, whether critical or not, it is always important to the individual.

Bioelectricity has been known at least since Galvani observed the effect of electrical current on frogs' legs nearly 200 years ago, and electrical activity has been noted in association with the heartbeat since 1856. In 1856, though, there was no way to characterize it, and what its clinical value might be was speculative at most. Its first useful graphic representation was the contribution of Augustus D. Waller in the 1880s. Waller, son of the English physiologist who described degeneration of nerve, was born in Paris, educated in Scotland, and worked in England. He had a long and illustrious career, but is remembered best for demonstrating that the electrical activity associated with the heartbeat can be recorded without opening the thorax, and that it precedes mechanical activity. He used a capillary electrometer in his experiments, a glass tube containing sulfuric acid in contact with mercury. The nature of this system is such that when there is change in the difference in electrical potential between its constituents their interface adjusts to reflect it. He connected the two ends of this device to the surface of the body and recorded the fluctuations of the mercury column on a moving photographic plate—the first human electrocardiogram.[24]

At about the time that Waller was working in London, another young man, a 27-year-old physiologist named Willem Einthoven, had begun his investigations of the same subject across the North Sea at the University of Leyden in Holland. He was dissatisfied with the response characteristics of the capillary electrometer and in 1903 published a description of a much more sensitive instrument.[25] The principle of his "string" galvanometer was simple; a movable conductor of electricity was suspended in the constant electrical field between the poles of a magnet so that, when a difference in potential between its two ends caused current to flow through it, setting up an electrical field about it, it deflected toward one pole or the other. When the two ends of the string were connected to the body, these deflections were a measure of the electrical activity of the heart. Einthoven used a strand of quartz plated with gold or platinum as the conductor/indicator, and recorded its motion by projecting its shadow on moving photographic film. Electronic amplification, and more effective recording systems, have evolved since Einthoven's time, but the method he devised is still the heart of all EKG machines.

Professor Einthoven also contributed more than anyone else to our understanding of the anatomic and physiologic characteristics of the body that govern the distribution of electrical signals at its surface, features that are approximately constant, and can be assumed to be true in humans generally, Einthoven's premises. These are the rules by which tracings are interpreted, and they are summarized as *Einthoven's triangle*, the original three leads (p. 86). In publications of early tracings made with capillary electrometers, the deflections were designated A, B, C, and D, but P, Q, R, S, T, and U were favored by Einthoven and, except for an early period of controversy, have been used ever since.[26, 570]

By 1910 or thereabouts the instrument for making tracings, the names of the waves, and the rules for interpreting them were in place, but the method was still mostly a laboratory oddity of interest to only physiologists. It was not long before its potential for the diagnosis of disease was recognized, though, and the first person associated prominently with clinical application was Sir Thomas Lewis. He was 28 years old when he became interested, and, four years later, in 1913, he wrote what was effectively the first textbook of electrocardiography.[701] One of Dr. Einthoven's friends, Dr. Samojloff, Professor of Physiology at the University of Kasan in Russia, had published one in 1909, but it was only 37 pages long, and, though written in German and published in Germany, its existence never became widely known. It was rediscovered recently by Dr. Krikler.[923]

Dr. Lewis knew Dr. Einthoven and cooperated with him, and with the Cambridge Instrument Company, in the development of methods and their application. He was interested chiefly in disorders of impulse formation and conduction, identified many of the principles that are the basis for modern practice, contrived much of the terminology, and is known best by today's medical students for

his application of electrocardiography to the study of "circus conduction" as an explanation for atrial fibrillation, an entity that had
been the subject of intense and productive study by Mackenzie using
recordings of jugular and apical pulses.

Electrocardiographers continued for a long time to be concerned
almost entirely with the formation and conduction of impulses, and
one reason for this was that so little was known of diseases affecting the structure and function of the ventricular myocardium.
Infarction had been recognized as a possibility in the late 19th century, but its identification as a clinical entity different from angina
pectoris dates from 1912 and the classic paper of James B. Herrick
of Chicago.[924] When his observations were presented to the Association of American Physicians, they aroused almost no interest at
all and went over "like a dud."[561] Herrick's interest continued,
though, and in 1917 he saw a 37-year-old doctor with chest pain,
and made an electrocardiogram that showed ST-T characteristics
similar to those that had been demonstrated in dogs following ligation of a coronary artery.[562] Thus began the use of the electrocardiogram in the diagnosis of myocardial infarction.

The ability of quinine to restore sinus mechanism in patients
with atrial fibrillation had been noted by Wenckebach, and in 1918
Frey introduced quinidine, an optical isomer of quinine and still the
prototype of antiarrhythmic agents.[576]

By 1920, then, myocardial infarction could be diagnosed, it was
possible to identify the disorders of impulse formation and conduction that may be associated with it, and potent antiarrhythmic therapy
was available, but there were not many EKG machines, and prominent cardiologists doubted the usefulness of the electrocardiogram.[575]
Texts published as late as the 1930s said almost nothing about
myocardial infarction, and it was not until the early 1940s that its
diagnosis became widespread.

Einthoven's original three leads were useful for study of forces
in the frontal plane only. In 1932 Wolferth and Wood suggested the
use of a postero-anterior lead, lead IV, made by placing the left arm
electrode on the back and the one from the right arm over the
precordium, and turning the selector switch to lead I.[28] This made a
tracing very similar to modern midprecordial leads but with the

polarity reversed. A modification, lead IVF, utilized the left arm electrode at the apex and the right arm electrode on the left leg to produce a curve with the polarity used today, but its accuracy and reproducibility were limited by the problem of defining the location of the apex. Also in 1932, Dr. Frank N. Wilson and his group published their first description of the central terminal of zero potential,[29] the basis for the V leads and three dimensional electrocardiography (pp. 88, 97), and the next few years saw a rapidly changing series of theories and lead systems.

In 1938 the American Heart Association and the Cardiac Society of Great Britain and Ireland did much to bring order to the field by agreeing on six positions for the chest electrode (designated by the letter C) defined in terms of easily identifiable bony landmarks, eliminating the need for locating the apex[30] (*see* p. 89). The same group agreed that the polarity of leads developed after the original three should be standardized with the "exploring" electrode positive. The position of the positive electrode determines the name of the lead, and a positive deflection during depolarization means that the electrical force is approaching that electrode (p. 78). IVF was replaced by leading from the several precordial positions to the right arm (CR), the left arm (CL), the left leg (CF), or Wilson's central terminal (V). There were differences of opinion as to the relative merits of these systems, but by the mid-1940s V leads were standard. Goldberger's "augmented" V leads followed very shortly (p. 88) and the lead system, in a state of flux for 15 years, became stable and has not changed since.

Experimental work, mostly with dogs, used leads with the exploring electrode applied directly to the epicardium, "direct" leads, and tracings from them were thought to be dominated by events in the tissue immediately subjacent to the electrode. When precordial leads were introduced, their proximity to the heart led to their being interpreted at first as "semidirect" leads. QRS patterns were seen as weighted by structures near their exploring electrodes, and there developed an elaborate system of explaining them by "rotation of the heart" when they were found in unusual positions. A qR pattern, for instance, seen commonly in V6, was attributed to depolarization of the IV septum to the right followed by the free wall of the ventricle to the left, and the same pattern seen in V1 with right ventricular hypertrophy was explained by rotation of the heart about its long axis so that V1 faced the surface normally seen by V6.[31] Each part of the heart does generate its own signals, but the nature of the galvanometer is such that all electrical information at any instant, from whatever source, is presented as a single point at a certain distance, and in a certain direction, from the zero point at the center of the system. The tracing is a continuum of these "instantaneous vectors."[14] There probably is some relation between habitus and orientation of the frontal QRS, the "vertical heart" of tall, thin people, and the "horizontal heart" of short, fat ones, but the idea of rotation of the heart to explain certain patterns, popular for a short time, was discredited long ago.[6, 7, 919, 925]

The only clinically important consequence of the proximity to the heart of the precordial leads is that the amplitude of the deflection due to a given force is greater in them than in the frontal ones. This means that the magnitude of spatial vectors cannot be calculated using frontal and precordial leads, but does not affect their direction, and magnitude is not often an important factor.

The limitations inherent in representation of all the electrical forces in the body as a single point on a line, a scalar value, were recognized early, and in 1920 Mann combined the information from two leads in a single figure that he called a monocardiogram.[55, 573] With development of the cathode ray oscilloscope in the 1920s,[574] it became possible to write this figure directly on a screen, a vectorcardiogram (VCG) (p. 90), but hope that substantial information not available in the scalar tracing could be had from this presentation proved to be unfounded; both methods show the same thing. Vectorcardiography is helpful in understanding the spatial relations of the twelve views, or leads, of the more convenient scalar tracing, but it is not well suited for analysis of time, and time is an important measurement, not only in relating events in the atria to those in the ventricles in a series of beats, but also those within a beat, and can be handled easily in a scalar tracing. Another limitation of vectorcardiography is that no reference frame for it has ever been accepted as standard. An equilateral tetrahedron would be a logical extension of Einthoven's triangle, but Einthoven's premises are not applicable in the postero-anterior dimension. The Frank system[477] has been used more than any other, but even that has been modified. There is no truly orthogonal system for electrocardiography, either scalar or vector, but leads I and aVF (X and Y, horizontal and vertical) are mutually perpendicular and define a frontal plane and, for practical purposes and within the clinical limits of the method, V1 serves effectively as a postero-anterior, or Z, lead. Lead systems are discussed in more detail in Chapter Five (p. 83).

The extreme sensitivity of the early string galvanometer that made it capable of recording tracings in the first place also made it very difficult to handle. Machines with better amplifiers and recorders were produced during the 1920s and 1930s, but these, too, were delicate, complicated, and expensive, and processing of exposed film was necessary before the tracing could be seen. In the 1940s, stable and dependable direct-writing systems were introduced, and, though there was some resistance to them on theoretically valid grounds, they soon replaced photographic methods. The most effective of these, a heated stylus writing on heat-sensitive paper, is still used, but is being replaced by a device known as a heat bar that writes by computer-controlled activation of two hundred or more dots-per-inch, each reacting instantaneously with specially prepared paper.

The technical capacity for making electrocardiograms at a distance was present from the beginning, Einthoven himself having recorded tracings from patients in a hospital a mile from his laboratory,[688] but there was little need for it before the 1950s. During that decade, means for electrical control of cardiac activity, pacing and defibrillation, were introduced, transmission of routine tracings by telephone became useful (p. 109), a profusion of monitoring devices appeared promptly, and the coronary care unit came into being.

By 1950 EKGs were available everywhere at low cost, but the process of extracting information from them still depended on rote memory and pattern recognition. At about that time, Dr. Robert P. Grant expressed some of the most basic principles of the method in terms that made it possible for doctors to relate tracings to what they had learned in medical school about anatomy and physiology. He emphasized the importance of understanding the temporal and spatial relation between ventricular depolarization and repolarization, and made this possible by a process he called "vector analysis" (p. 30). This did not eliminate the value of experience and judgment in interpretation, but made patterns more meaningful by showing their derivation, much as patterns are recognized by physical diagnosis. Dr. Grant's work was a major development in the history of electrocardiography, and any serious student of the subject must be familiar with it.[14,956,957]

While all these advances in understanding and instrumentation were being introduced, interpretation of tracings by methods that had been used since the beginning of the century continued. Qualified doctors were few and "reading" of EKGs was a small component of their work; detailed analysis of the curves, necessary for secure interpretation, was simply too tedious to be practical. With the advent of the digital computer in the 1960s, this conflict between what should be done and what could be done began to be resolved.

Machines can be classified as *prosthetic*, those that do only what humans can do but do it faster or better, and *autonomous*, those that do things that humans cannot do under any circumstances, as, for instance, a clock.[572] A digital computer is a prosthetic device in this sense, ideally suited for manipulation of data such as those in scalar electrocardiograms after they have been converted to numbers; it can do purely mechanical "scut work," whereas a human's brain is used for thinking, for making decisions. It offers much help to the electrocardiographer but, as with all new techniques, introduces new dangers as well, chiefly the risk that its limitations will not be understood and that its product may be accepted as an interpretation (p. 224).

What of the future? Einthoven called the graph he produced an elektrokardiogramm, EKG. The E has been subdivided, and we now have scalar and vector presentations, but, even when the data from planes perpendicular to each other are correlated to produce information in three dimensions, only a series of net values is represented, and neither the vector concept nor computer-assisted analysis changes this. At least in theory, the future must hold a holocardio-gram, a three-dimensional image that can be viewed from any angle, much as a sculpture. To produce such a figure would require a technique for adapting the signals available at the surface of the body for reproduction by holographic methods. This has not been done yet, but it is tempting to predict the result applied to ventricular depolarization, a kind of a three-dimensional figure that could show, literally, electrical holes in the heart.[926]

FOUR

Anatomic and Physiologic Basis of the Electrocardiogram

It is assumed that the reader is familiar with the anatomy and physiology of the normal heart, but a summary of some features with direct bearing on electrocardiography is in order.

The *sinus node*, a structure defined only vaguely in the morphologic sense, is an aggregation of specialized tissue in the right atrial wall near the superior vena cava[536] (Fig. 4-1). It is the pacemaker for the normal heartbeat, generating impulses at the rate of between about 40 and 140/min. Each impulse sets in motion a wavefront of electrical activity that advances circumferentially over the atria, like ripples spreading from a stone dropped in a pond, at a rate of about *1000 mm/s*, activating the right atrium first, continuing into the left, and converging at the AV node. There are pathways of preferential conduction between the sinus and AV nodes, but these are not of clinical importance, and it is the atrial wall, a curved plane with no thickness from an electrical point of view,[33-36] over which the impulse moves.

The *AV node*, an ovoid structure about 5 mm long,[38] lies in the base of the interatrial septum near the coronary sinus and is the only electrical connection between atria and ventricles. It has the slowest rate of conduction in the whole intracardiac conduction system, about *twenty millimeters/s*, forming the spout of an electrical funnel (p. 121) and limiting the number of impulses that can be conducted to the ventricles to about 180–200/min.

Leaving the node, the impulse enters the specialized conduction tissue of the *Bundle of His*,[412, 507] which extends into the superior aspect of the IV septum and conducts very rapidly, up to *4000 mm/s*. This structure is composed of multiple interlacing longitudinal pathways and divides in the superior aspect of the interventricular septum into a small, clearly defined right branch and a relatively

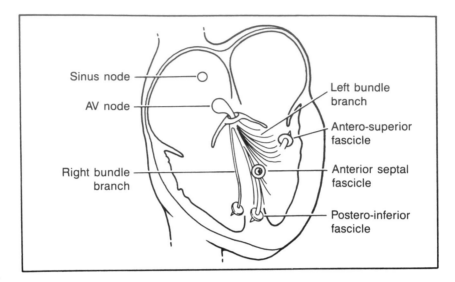

Fig. 4-1. A diagram of the intracardiac system.

large, diffuse left one. The *right branch* continues as a thin, undivided strand down the right side of the interventricular septum and through the moderator band to the anterior papillary muscle of the right ventricle, after which its branching is widespread. The anatomy of the *left branch*, less clearly defined and subject to much more interpretation, can be compared to a cable in contrast to the wire of the right branch. Early in its course, in the subendocardial aspect of the left side of the interventricular septum just beneath the aortic valve, it divides into more or less well-defined groups, or fascicles, of fibers, anterior, posterior, and septal. There is some question as to whether these are functionally distinct, but it is widely accepted that they are (p. 161).

The impulse is propagated so rapidly in this system that, in effect, it reaches the whole subendocardial surface of *both ventricles* at the same time. Neither the anatomy nor the physiology of what happens next is perfectly clear, but it is probable that fibers of specialized conduction tissue, the His-Purkinje system, continue into the inner part, perhaps two-thirds, of the wall, and that signals generated there are in random directions at very rapid rates, effectively canceling each other. There are conflicting interpretations of this process, but the weight of evidence is that events in the inner part of the wall cannot be identified in the surface tracing. However thick this zone may be, there is at some level an "electrical endocardium"[927] outside which the process is propagated through the myocardium itself the rest of the way to the epicardium at a rate of only about *400 mm/s*.[227, 725, 728, 928]

Now consider the ventricular myocardium as if it were a hollow ball with its wall of equal thickness and the impulse proceeding outward from the center.[928] Forces in opposite directions would be equal, canceling each other, and no deflection at all would be recorded by a galvanometer set up to observe the process. Modify this hypothetical system by inserting a septum across the cavity of the ball and depolarizing it simultaneously from both sides toward its center. These forces, occurring at the same time that the free walls are being activated, also cancel out, and the result is still nothing. This model is a good starting point because it is easy to see, and it is easy to make the jump from it to what is known of the anatomy and physiology of the human heart. The idea of simultaneous radial depolarization is valid, things really work that way, and the hypothetical model of the IV septum as described is, too, at least in a general way, because the IV septum is related embryologically to both ventricles, and forces generated in it, directed outward from the endocardium, oppose each other. The ventricular myocardium is not symmetrical, though, or even a closed system; its right-upper-posterior limit is the mitral and tricuspid valves, and no electrical forces are generated there. The thickness of the ventricular walls, and of the IV septum, varies widely, and so does the relative amount of the septum embryologically related to the right and left ventricles; the sum of the forces at play at any instant during ventricular depolarization is not the same in all hearts.

The left ventricular mass is much greater than the right, and the net result of their simultaneous depolarization, over a period of about 0.08 s, is a complex of curves directed, as a whole, to the left, caudad, and usually dorsad. The process is sometimes initiated by a tiny force directed opposite the principal one, and this has been called a *septal Q*. When it is recognized that the galvanometer reduces all forces to a single point, though, and that the IV septum lies substantially in the frontal plane of the body, to interpret this wave as evidence of activity in the septum specifically has "little validity."[7]

The *electrophysiology of the cell* is basic to all the events just described. Living muscle cells in the resting state are polarized. Each is surrounded by what amounts to an insulating membrane with positive charges on the outside balanced by negative ones on the inside. The potential difference across this membrane is of the order of eighty millivolts, but it is not detectable by a galvanometer both of whose electrodes are outside the cell. When a stimulus effectively punctures this shield, removing the insulation between opposing forces, the potential difference between them is open to the "volume conductor" of the surrounding medium and can be recorded by a galvanometer whose electrodes are at a distance.

A few diagrams can help. Figure 4-2 represents a muscle cell, or a strip of muscle, in a volume conductor observed from the positive *(exploring)* pole of a unipolar lead. In the resting, or polarized, state (A), no difference of potential is apparent from the outside. The indicator registers zero and writes a flat line when paper is drawn past it. When the membrane is rendered permeable to electrical charges at the end of the strip farthest from the electrode, the polarized state cannot be maintained—positive and negative charges are no longer neatly arranged in an equal and opposite fashion; the tissue at the point of stimulus is not polarized, but, for the instant, the rest of it still is. A boundary of potential difference now exists, and proceeds away from this point with its leading edge positive and its trailing edge negative. As this approaches the positive pole of a lead, its progress is recorded as an upstroke (B and C). Stated differently, an upward deflection of the trace means that the positive pole of the lead faces the positive side of a boundary of potential difference; a negative deflection, the negative side. When the whole strip has been depolarized (D), there is no potential difference in the system, and the trace returns to the level that indicates this, zero.

Soon, repolarization begins at the same point at which depolarization had begun, reestablishing a boundary of potential difference, but this time with reversed polarity (E), its negative side now

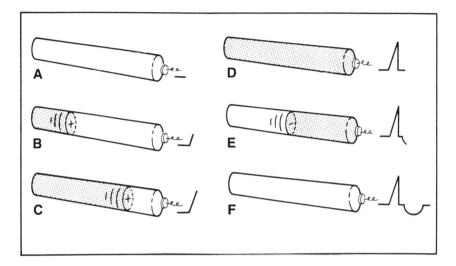

Fig. 4-2. Depolarization and repolarization of a hypothetical muscle strip.

facing the positive pole of the lead. It takes longer to store up energy than it does to release it, and the curve that represents this part of the cycle is longer than both that of depolarization and of opposite sign. In this hypothetical example, the energy stored equals that released, and the areas of the two curves are equal (F).

Energy conversion in the beating heart, however, is not 100% efficient, and the curves representing its depolarization and repolarization are not equal and opposite. How far they depart from this ideal is one of the things that define normal *(see below)*. The release of energy, represented in the tracing by QRS, is relatively massive and stable, not modified easily. Its restoration, represented by ST-T, is a slower process producing smaller potentials and can be altered by almost any change in its environment, e.g., temperature, pressure, and chemical factors.

Consider Fig. 4-3. Depolarization and repolarization are represented as in Fig. 4-2, but with the hypothesis that there is a physiologic gradient of some kind, maximal at the left end of the strip and minimal at the right, indicated by the device added above. Depolarization (A, B, C) has not been changed detectably, but the gradi-

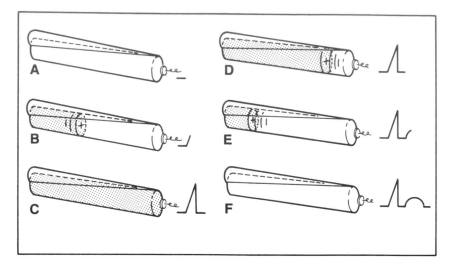

Fig. 4-3. Effect of transmyocardial gradients on repolarization.

ent has prolonged the refractory period of the tissue at the left of the strip so that repolarization now proceeds from right to left, backing away from the electrode, as it were, still presenting its positive face and writing a positive curve (D, E, F).

This example is extremely simplistic, of course, but serves to express the idea of what happens. In the myocardium of the beating heart, there are multiple gradients from endocardium to epicardium,[405] gradients of oxygen, lactic acid, temperature, and pressure, for instance. The course of repolarization is influenced by all of these, and the result is curves, in V6, for instance, similar to those in the diagram. Instead of being opposite each other, the orientation of the curve written by repolarization is close to that of depolarization. The spatial relation between them is called the *ventricular gradient*, something not often calculated, but a concept used in every interpretation for integration of the information displayed during repolarization with that of depolarization (p. 52).[14,45–49, 449, 853, 855, 919]

Whatever other factors may be at work, the course of recovery is influenced by that of excitation;[48,50] if the ventricles are activated over a route other than normal, the course by which potential is restored must be altered accordingly (p. 201). Think of the record of repolarization as a chart of the course taken by a water skier, and the depolarization curve as the boat. The skier must follow the boat in a general way but does not have to duplicate its course precisely. If the track taken by the skier crisscrosses the wake of the boat as it takes a "normal" course across the lake, it describes a primary abnormality; if it follows exactly behind the boat while the boat pursues an erratic course, the "abnormality" is secondary. It is possible, of course, for both primary and secondary abnormalities to be present at the same time, but this is difficult to recognize.

The anatomic and physiologic features considered so far are central to generation of the curves recorded in an electrocardiogram, but the tracing is a remote and imprecise representation of them, influenced by many factors outside the heart. (*See* Einthoven's premises, p. 85.)

FIVE

Lead Systems

An electrocardiogram is a chart of the course through space and time of a point as it departs from another, fixed, point and returns to it. The direction it moves, how far, and at what rate determine the amplitude, sign, duration, and contour of the curves representing its projection on the various leads, and correlation of these curves with health or disease has given them clinical usefulness. The events they reflect occur in three dimensions, and a three-dimensional reference frame is necessary for their measurement. Without agreement as to how left and right, up and down, and front and back, as well time and amplitude, are to be defined, and their parts coordinated, the tracing, like the elephant in John Godfrey Saxe's poem, would be subject to as many descriptions and interpretations as there are observers.

The Blind Men and the Elephant

It was six men of Indostan
   To learning much inclined,
Who went to see the Elephant
   (Though all of them were blind),
That each by observation
Might satisfy his mind.

The First approached the Elephant,
And happening to fall
Against his broad and sturdy side,
At once began to bawl:
"God bless me! But the Elephant
Is very like a wall!"

The Second, feeling of the tusk,
Cried, "Ho! What have we here

So very round and smooth and sharp?
To me 'tis mighty clear
This wonder of an Elephant
Is very like a spear!"

The Third approached the animal,
And happening to take
The squirming trunk within his hands,
Thus boldly up and spake:
"I see," quoth he, "the Elephant
Is very like a snake!"

The Fourth reached out an eager hand,
And felt about the knee.
"What most this beast is like
Is mighty plain," quoth he;
"Tis clear enough the Elephant
Is very like a tree!"

The fifth, who chanced to touch the ear,
said: "E'en the blindest man
Can tell what this resembles most;
Deny the fact who can,
This marvel of an Elephant
Is very like a fan!"

The sixth no sooner had begun
About the beast to grope,
Than, seizing on the swinging tail
That fell within his scope,
"I see," quoth he, "the Elephant
Is very like a rope!"

And so these men of Indostan
Disputed loud and long,
Each in his own opinion
Exceeding stiff and strong,
Though each was partly in the right,
And all were in the wrong!

    The Moral:

> So oft in theologic wars,
> The disputants, I ween,
> Rail on in utter ignorance
> Of what each other mean,
> And prat about an Elephant
> Not one of them has seen!

An electrocardiogram is very like an elephant in a box. Assume you have never seen an elephant, but that there is one before you in a big box. One way to find our what it looks like is to bore holes in the box; bore three, and label them I, II, and III (Fig. 5-1). A forehead is seen through number I, a side through II, and a tail through III. This is a normal elephant. Go away for a while, then come back, and find that you see a tail through I, a side through II, and a forehead through III. Depending strictly on patterns, the elephant must now be classified as abnormal; it is different from what was defined as normal. You know better, though; the elephant has just turned around in the box. If there were to be a forehead, tail, and side in I, II, and III, there really would be something wrong, but this is evident only because, contrary to the initial assumption, you do know what an elephant looks like—and that elephants are normal or abnormal according to how they are put together and compare to other elephants. Their position in space is considered in describing them, whether standing up or lying down, facing east or facing west, but this is not often critical in defining abnormality.

The analogy is obvious. The box is the body, the elephant represents the anatomy and physiology of the heart as expressed in the electrocardiogram, and the holes are the leads, or views. Like an elephant, an electrocardiogram has several parts that can be described separately and coordinated with others. Patterns learned empirically are helpful, but if we understand how they came to be that way their value is enhanced, and variants can be dealt with more confidently.

Fortunately, there are universally accepted standards for recognizing the three dimensions, and for plotting time on the horizontal scale and amplitude (voltage) on the vertical one. They are based on Einthoven's premises, published in 1913,[930] and these can be summarized usefully as follows:

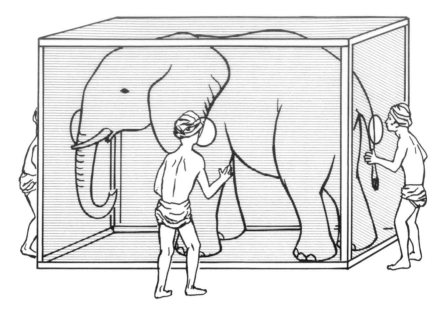

Fig. 5-1. An elephant in a box.

1. The heart acts as a single dipole, i.e., a very small generator;
2. It is located in the center of a homogeneous volume conductor; and
3. It is equidistant from the shoulders and symphysis pubis.

These are expressed graphically as *Einthoven's triangle* (Fig. 5-2). The difference in potential between the left and right upper apices, shown when the positive pole of the galvanometer is attached to the left arm and the negative one to the right arm, is called Lead I. The inferior apex can be represented by either leg, but the left is the one that is used, and, when this is positive and the right arm negative, the connection is called Lead II. For Lead III, the left leg is positive and the left arm negative. These are still referred to sometimes as the *standard*, or *bipolar*, leads, but a routine tracing now includes three additional leads in the frontal plane and six in the horizontal, and the nature of a galvanometer makes it necessary for any lead to have two connections to the body.

The volume conductor named in the premises is composed of thorax and abdomen, with the arms and legs acting as linear con-

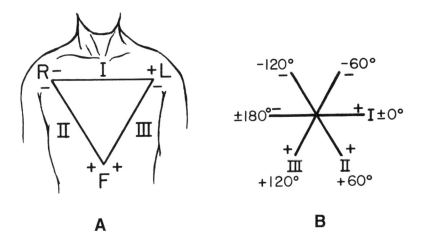

Fig. 5-2. Einthoven's triangle (**A**) and the same information expressed as a triaxial reference system (**B**). *See* p. 86.

ductors, wires, attached to the body at the shoulders and symphysis pubis. Numerous alternative reference systems have been proposed, but none has lasted, and Einthoven's premises still underlie the practice of electrocardiography. They are so fundamental, so accepted, that it is often simply assumed that everyone understands them, and they are not even mentioned, kind of like Magritte's picture of a pipe with a label that says "this is not a pipe." It is a *picture* of a pipe, of course, and the title assumes everyone knows that. It is important to identify one's assumptions so that they can be tested, especially when actions based on them make a difference to the patient; if one is not valid, adjustments must be made in reasoning to reflect this.

Adding the Third Dimension

Early in the development of lead systems it was realized that it would be more logical to measure the difference in potential between a point on the body and the zero point at the center of the system, a single unknown, than that between two unknowns on the surface, but it was thought that this could not be achieved. The validity of the frontal lead system rests on the assumption that the shoulders and symphysis pubis are equidistant from each other and from the heart, and human anatomy is such that no point on the anterior or posterior wall of the chest is nearly so far from the heart as these three. In 1932, though, Dr. Wilson and his associates at the University of Michigan, building on Einthoven's work, constructed a lead system that does define a point whose electrical potential does not vary during the cardiac cycle (Fig. 5-3A), and can be used as a fixed reference. The circuitry is based on Kirchoff's fist law, which says that the algebraic sum of the electrical potentials in a closed network of wires is zero, circumstances satisfied by connecting all three corners of Einthoven's triangle at a point. A lead utilizing this *central terminal of zero potential* as its negative pole is for practical purposes a truly *unipolar* lead,[32] measuring the difference between it and a point on the surface of the body. Leads using this method are called V leads (V for voltage). *See* p. 97.

The Wilson system promptly became standard for precordial leads but produced such small complexes when applied in the frontal plane, VR, VL, and VF, that interpretation was difficult. In 1942 Emanuel Goldberger, in New York, suggested a modification. He noted that, when the central terminal was used for leads from the three corners of the triangle, the potential at an extremity is delivered to both sides of the galvanometer, as part of the central terminal defining the negative pole, and, through the exploring electrode, to the positive one, and reasoned that, if the connection to the central terminal were interrupted, the complexes recorded would be half again as large as VR, VL, and VF, but that their configuration would not change. Mathematical proof of this hypothesis is relatively simple and is stated clearly by Goldberger in his text.[31] The complexes obtained by this modification are called *augmented* unipolar limb leads: aVR, aVL, and aVF, and fit easily into the Einthoven triangle to make a hexaxial reference system with 30° between lines (Fig. 5-3B). A given change in voltage does not produce the same amplitude of deflection in augmented leads as in leads I, II, and III, but this is not often important.

Einthoven's premises imply that leads I and aVF are perpendicular to each other, defining horizontal and vertical dimensions, the frontal plane, and the validity of this can be demonstrated easily

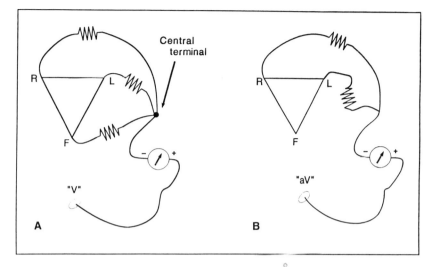

Fig. 5-3. **(A)** Wilson's central terminal of zero potential for V leads; **(B)**, Goldberger's modification for augmented V leads.

in the process of describing only a few tracings. No lead is as accurately perpendicular to the frontal plane as Leads I and aVF are to each other, but Vl works so well for this purpose, within the clinical limits of the method, that there has been little interest in improving on it since Frank's efforts in the 1950s.[477] Leads I and V1 define a horizontal plane effectively perpendicular to the frontal one. Pragmatically, then, Leads I, aVF, and V1 provide an effectively orthogonal reference system for three dimensions (Fig. 2-3).

The figure for the horizontal plane used on the worksheet (and in Fig. 5-4) is not so routine as the hexaxial schema for the frontal one, and much less precise, but helpful.[57, 58] The angle between adjacent precordial leads is assumed to be 20°, and, in practice, V1 is regarded as perpendicular to the frontal plane. The positions for six chest leads are standard, and are located with reference to easily identifiable bony landmarks (p. 97).[30]

All leads view the processes of depolarization and repolarization as if the whole heart were equally remote from the exploring electrode,[925] and all show the whole. No lead is better than any other except as its view of the event in question may be more effective.

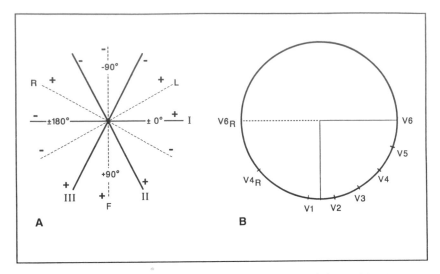

Fig. 5-4. Reference figures for frontal plane (**A**), and horizontal plane (**B**).

Vectorcardiography

A value that has only magnitude can be represented by a number, a point on a scale, and is called a *scalar*; one that has both magnitude and direction, represented by a line, is called a *vector*. When a vector symbolizes a force, a third quality, the heading, polarity, or sense, is indicated by adding a point at one end. When the electrical activity of the heart was first documented, the only method of recording it was scalar, producing graphs of the projection of a moving point (p. 86) on three lines, leads I, II, and III. The idea of plotting two leads simultaneously as a two-dimensional, or vector, figure, and a little later the technology to do this electronically, developed in the 1920s (p. 70), and vectorcardiography was born. Both forms are electrocardiograms, of course, but *EKG* (or *ECG*) still refers to the scalar form; a vectorcardiogram is called a *VCG*.

It was hoped at first that vectorcardiography would offer information not available from the EKG, but they both represent exactly the same unknown, and the scalar form makes it much more acces-

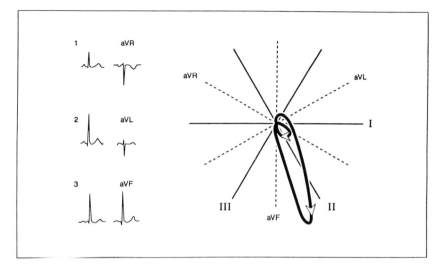

Fig. 5-5. Scalar and vector presentations of the same information.

sible than the vector, mostly because it is difficult to separate the subdivisions of the tracing in the vector presentation, and to relate the timing of events in one beat to those in others; also, no reference frame for the anteroposterior dimension has become standard. Use of a loop to represent the view of the unknown from two leads at the same time has great value, however, as a tool to demonstrate the spatial interrelation of the leads.[55,56,956]

Figure 5-5 shows a frontal plane scalarcardiogram, or routine EKG, and the vectorcardiogram derived from its leads I and III. Pick a point on the QRS loop, say the one at its greatest distance from the center, and drop imaginary perpendiculars to the I and III lines. The values will be positive in both leads, greater in III than I. Now drop perpendiculars from the same or any other point to other leads and note how accurately you have predicted the scalar tracing. Practice reversing this process, constructing a VCG from two leads of an EKG and deriving the others. It is easier if the tracing is made at 50 mm/s and double gain, but reassuring figures can be drawn using only a routine tracing. Einthoven's premises work.

Six

Electrocardiographic Equipment and Methods

INCLUDING ARTIFACTS AND TECHNICAL ERRORS

We think of an electrocardiogram as representing electrical activity in the heart, of course, and it does, but that may not be all; the heart is not the only organ in the body that produces electricity. The brain generates voltages too, and so do muscles and the fetal heart, and differences in potential may arise at the skin–electrode interface. In addition, both patient and recording equipment may act as antennae to detect the electrical field, alternating 60 times/s in a polarity, that is almost ubiquitous in our environment. The position of the trace at any moment represents the net of all these, not just information from the heart. Factors other than electricity can influence the tracing, too, especially the skill, attention, and understanding of the technician. A lead labeled II, for instance, is really III if it was made with the arm leads crossed, I if the left arm and leg leads were transposed, and contains no information at all if the right arm lead was attached to the right leg and vice versa (p. 104), and all these human errors are common. Deflections caused by extracardiac activity or technical error are called artifacts, and may arise in any part of the system—the patient's body, the recording equipment, computers, facsimile machines, and telephone lines.

Signals from the brain and fetal heart are so small and remote that they are not a problem, skeletal muscle activity can usually be controlled to acceptable levels (p. 102), the problem of sixty-cycle artifact, a major one until very recently, has been all but eliminated by advances in technology (pp. 99, 102), and artifacts originating in other parts of the system are relatively uncommon. Most can be recognized easily, either by the technician as the tracing is being

93

made, or by the doctor later, but unrecognized they can mean real trouble. Their largest source by far is human error, and both doctors and technicians must remain on the alert for them. Most doctors have not recorded many tracings themselves, and the training of most technicians has been by coworkers, or in radiology or respiratory therapy, and has included little instruction about galvanometers, grounding, lead systems, and electrocardiographic theory.[375–379,777,778] The observations in this chapter are those of a clinician whose experience has sensitized him to the problem. They are not very technical, but include points that can be of help to both technicians and those who supervise their work and interpret its product. The goal is to enhance the potential value, and minimize the risk, of having an electrocardiogram made.

The EKG Machine

As a processor of electromagnetic information, an EKG machine is a lot like a radio. Each has three stages: an apparatus for collecting minuscule electrical signals, an amplifier to make them large enough to work with, and a device for changing them into another form. The patient cable of an EKG machine compares to the antenna of a radio, and the recorder to the speaker.

There are two types of EKG machines, analog and digital. *Analog machines* detect the continuously variable electrical activity in the heart, amplify it, and record it while it is in progress. *Digital machines* convert the information to digits, or numbers, first, store these in a computer, analyze them, then retrieve them and reproduce the tracing, events that explain the lag between acquisition of data and production of the tracing. Data acquired by analog machines can be digitized and analyzed by computers in a separate step, but computers are not integral parts of them.

Most machines made now are digital, but there are many analog ones still in service, and both are discussed in the pages that follow. Even very old machines, properly maintained, can produce satisfactory tracings, but maintenance becomes more and more of a problem; one of the principal advantages of current models is that they require minimal maintenance. Doctors and technicians do not need to understand all the physics and engineering involved, but they are responsible for proper use of the equipment and should know at least what each component of the system contributes to the product.

Kirchoff's first law states that the sum of all the potentials in a closed network at any instant is zero, and *Einthoven's law* relates this to the frontal electrocardiogram by noting that at any instant, the sum of the values in Lead I and Lead III equals that in Lead II— "I plus III equals II." This is also fundamental to data acquisition in digital equipment. The machine acquires the precordial leads individually, but only two frontal ones, constructing the other four from them. If the connection to an arm or the left leg is defective, a frontal lead that includes that apex of the triangle will be off the chart with an analog machine. With digital equipment, though, a flat line is recorded in the augmented unipolar lead involved (aVR, aVL, or aVF), and, though a tracing appears in the other two, it is not valid; in the *bipolar* leads (I, II, and III), the one that does not include the defective connection is unaffected, but the (mirror image) curves that appear in the other two are artifactual.

The *recorder* consists of a paper transport mechanism and a stylus, or other form of movable point, for writing. The characteristics of the paper and the writing point vary, but in almost every case sensitized paper is required; in very few is ink simply applied to plain paper. The most popular current method uses thermal paper that changes color when heated. This is drawn past a "heat bar," or thermal dot printer, with 200–300 independent dots per inch (DPI), each of which can be switched on and off instantaneously by a computer reading from stored data. This system produces a clean line without the mechanical problems that plague writers dependent on moving pens; the paper transport mechanism is its only moving part.

Analog machines write by means of a stylus moving in an arc of a circle and incorporating various devices produce straight lines, "rectilinear conversion." Most utilize heated elements to melt the colored covering on special paper and leave a black line, either a pointed stylus in contact with the paper as it is passes over a flat surface, or a ribbon stylus touching the paper at only one point as it is drawn over a sharp edge. Still others use special nozzles and inks, and jets, electrostatic methods, and various forms of carbon transfer have been used also. The manual that comes with the machine will describe its writing system and give instructions for first echelon maintenance. Details vary widely. Equipment continues to be refined, made more versatile and dependable, but all EKG machines still employ the principles introduced by Professor Einthoven nearly a hundred years ago (p. 85).

Preparation of the Patient

Tracings are made routinely with the patient supine to minimize skeletal muscle activity, the most common source of unwanted potentials, but they can be made in any position when necessary. Relaxation can be helped by a few words of explanation and reassurance, and a pillow or a blanket.

With the machine turned on and ready to go, a small amount of electrode jelly is applied at each electrode site and rubbed gently into the skin. The purpose of this is to minimize skin resistance and provide good electrical continuity between the patient and the recording equipment *(see below)*. Reduction of skin resistance is not nearly so critical as it was before very strong signals could be provided by amplification, but it is still important in the interests of consistency and stability. Care should be taken in preparation of sites for precordial leads, using only a minimal amount of jelly. If the area prepared for one overlaps that for the next, the result is as if one big electrode covered both areas, and detail in the tracing may be blurred.[501] Disposable electrodes eliminate the need for site preparation, and are convenient and widely used, but expensive and not necessary.

It makes no difference where on an arm or a leg an electrode is placed, because the arms and legs are linear conductors, extensions of the patient cable, connected to the trunk at the shoulders and the symphysis pubis. If suction electrodes are used, those for the arms may be attached to the anterior aspect of the shoulders; if plate electrodes are held by straps, it is best to apply them over soft tissues to insure good contact with their whole surface—high on the volar aspect of the forearms, and the inner aspect of the calves, are the usual places. The straps should be just tight enough to hold the electrodes on comfortably; if they are tight enough to cause discomfort, or loose enough to slip, artifacts (wandering baseline or muscle tremor) may result. If an arm is missing, the electrode can be attached to the body at the shoulder. Either or both of the leg electrodes can be attached to either leg, since both are in continuity with the body at the same point, the inferior angle of Einthoven's triangle, the symphysis pubis. Remember, the right leg electrode is for grounding (p. 99) and does not enter directly into the tracing; it will work wherever it is attached to the body.

The positions for precordial leads are critical, and are shown in Fig. 6-1. Common usage suggests that *V1* is a position, and that the precordial leads are the *V leads*. This is not really a problem, but what *V* defines is use of Wilson's central electrode of zero potential (p. 88) as the negative pole of a lead, not the position of the positive, or exploring, electrode. The numbers identify positions on the chest for the exploring electrode and were designated originally by the letter C; before V leads came into universal use, we had CR, CL, and CF leads (p. 69). The chest positions are nonnegotiable and are defined as follows: #1, fourth intercostal space just to the right of the sternum; #2, fourth intercostal space just to the left of the sternum; #3, halfway between 2 and 4; #4, fifth intercostal space at the left midclavicular line; #5, the same horizontal level as 4 (i.e., parallel to the floor if the patient were standing) in the left anterior axillary line; and #6, the same level in the left midaxillary line.

Leads made at corresponding positions on the right side of the chest are marked with the suffix "R"—V3R, V4R, V5R, and V6R (positions 1 and 2 do not change names). VE is at the ensiform cartilage, V7 is in the left posterior axillary line at the same horizontal level as V6, and V8 is in the midscapular line. Tracings may be recorded from other points, but when this is done their positions must be indicated. Note that the nomenclature and positioning of electrodes are the same whether the patient has dextrocardia or not. If a position is inaccessible, e.g., bandage, chest tube, that lead must be omitted.

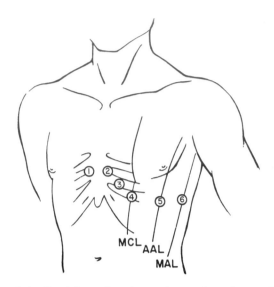

Fig. 6-1. Positions for chest electrodes. *See* p. 97.

Calibration

A reference value for amplitude is to the EKG what a scale of miles is to a road map, and from the very beginning of the method this has been standard: One millivolt produces a deflection of ten millimeters; voltages are always corrected to this standard, and documentation of it is the calibration. When QRS is so large that it runs off the chart, the scale can be halved. It makes little difference what amplification (gain) is used, as long as the curves are big enough to be seen and the calibration is recorded, but recording at half gain, except when QRS is too large to fit on the chart, obscures detail. Most machines offer the option of automatic switching to half gain for precordial leads only. There is almost never any benefit to be had from recording at double gain; everything is doubled equally, and discrimination is not enhanced. It is like writing very large for someone who can't read.

The calibration pulse documents, not only the amplitude of the deflection produced by one millivolt, but also frequency response and paper speed. Its corners should be sharp and square. If the stylus is overdamped, pressing too hard on the paper, the corners will be rounded, indicating inadequate response to high frequencies; if underdamped, too little pressure, there will be overshoot. Clinically important errors of interpretation may result from overdamping,[381-383] especially ST depression simulating the picture of coronary insufficiency. Inappropriate damping is not a problem with digital equipment. The duration of calibration is exactly 0.2 s, documenting paper speed (p. 104).

Labeling the Tracing

The patient's name and identification number, as well as the date and time it was recorded, and, when the technology permits, the name of the technician, must be noted on every tracing; an unidentified tracing is worse in some ways than no tracing at all. Most machines now on the market provide keys for entering numbers and letters, and take care of date and time automatically, but human error, perhaps just a wrong keystroke, is still a possibility with potentially serious consequences. Automatic labeling of leads assumes that the patient cable connections, and positions of electrodes on the body, are all correct, that the lead plugged into the V2 slot in the data acquisition unit, for instance, is from an electrode in the fourth intercostal space just to the left of the sternum; if it is not, and if the doctor assumes that it is, the patient may be hurt.

Grounding, Electrical Hazards, 60-Cycle Artifact

There is some risk of shock in working with any electrical equipment, 60-cycle artifact is still occasionally an annoyance, and the chance of both is reduced by proper grounding. Grounding is an important concept that can be illustrated by comparing electricity to water power.

The evaporation of water, its condensation, falling as rain, and its return to the sea, an endless cycle powered by the sun, is understood by everyone, and it is easy to see how falling water turns wheels and performs work. Electricity works in almost exactly the same way. It cannot be seen or heard or felt, but is a fundamental force in nature that, like gravity, can be used without being completely understood.

Mechanical energy (falling water) can be converted to electrical energy by being made to turn generators that separate elementary particles, protons and electrons. The tendency of these to return to their undisturbed state is called electricity, and the energy it represents can be channeled through wires, much as water is channeled through pipes as it seeks its lowest level, flowing from levels of higher potential to lower, "turning the wheels" of whatever device is set in its path. Its power, or potential, is expressed in volts; volts (above "ground," or zero) are to electricity what feet above sea level are to water power. In the electrical systems that power our lights, TV sets, and EKG machines, the energy is carefully kept within its channels by insulation, just as water is contained within pipes, so that its flow can be directed.

When two objects with different electrical values come close enough to each other to permit it, a current flows between them until the difference is canceled; lightning is an example. There is a chance that differences in potential may develop between parts of an electrical system with the risk of producing unwanted currents or *short circuits*. In order to minimize this risk, all conductive parts of the supporting framework, or chassis, of the system are insulated from the power supply and connected to each other, creating a relatively large *electron exchanger* and preventing buildup of potential in any one part with relation to others. The ultimate electron exchanger, the unchanging zero reference for all electrical systems, is the world itself, the earth, or ground. In a sense, the theoretical center of the system, the B point, is the *ground* for interpreting the tracing.

When the word is used literally, to *ground* something means to make an electrical connection between it and the earth, *true ground*, but it is used also in a more restricted sense. The chassis of an electrical device, serving as an electron exchanger for that device alone, is called a *chassis ground*, and, when two or more devices operate within a system, they can be connected to provide a *system ground*. The third prong of the power supply in most hospitals provides an additional connection between the chassis of the instrument and the earth itself at some nearby point, and the commercial network includes many points where its supports are grounded in order to prevent differences in potential during transmission.

Two characteristics of the 110–120 volt power supply standard in the United States are relevant: it reverses its polarity sixty times a second (60-cycle alternating current, or 60 Hertz AC), and it broadcasts a signal in its vicinity. Both the EKG machine and the patient's body act as antennae and receive this signal. In recording a tracing, the only potentials we want to see are those that originate in the heart, and, as long as the body and the galvanometer are influenced equally by the 60-cycle signal, these are all we do see, but, if the efficiency of the body-antenna is not the same as that of the machine-antenna, the difference between them shows in the tracing, oscillating sixty times a second. Connecting the "chassis of the heart" to the chassis of the galvanometer, via the right leg lead, forms a system ground and precludes a difference in potential between its two components. The position of the data acquisition unit in the patient cable very close to the patient helps by shortening the lead wires.

Antennae other than the patient and the EKG machine may be encountered. The bed, other equipment, or another person in contact with the patient may serve as sources of AC interference that can be eliminated by breaking the connection or by grounding the offending antenna to the EKG machine. The instructions in the user's manual that came with the machine may identify other possibilities, and sometimes a little detective work is necessary to localize the problem.

There is almost no hazard to either patient or technician in recording an electrocardiogram with properly maintained equipment when the patient is not connected to another line-powered device at the same time, but if there is such a connection, to a monitor for instance, and the potential-to-ground is not exactly the same for both this and the EKG machine, the difference between them will cause a current to flow through the patient's body. In the rare instance in which this occurs, the density of the electrical field in the area of the heart will usually be so small that it will not be significant, but if there is a low-resistance pathway into the patient's heart, a saline filled catheter for instance, in continuity with electrical equipment with a potential-to-ground different from that of the EKG machine, the current density in the myocardium may be great enough to induce ventricular fibrillation. The use of monitors and electric beds has increased this kind of risk to the patient as well as the operator.[380,396] When recording a tracing from a patient who is connected to other equipment, the other equipment should be disconnected from the power supply—unplugged, not just turned off—before the patient is connected to the EKG machine, and neither patient nor technician should touch another electrically powered device.

Baseline Artifacts

Muscle tremor (Fig. 6-2B) produces random motion of the stylus with spiking, high-frequency deflections of varying amplitude, "noise" as compared to the smoother and generally smaller *f* waves of atrial fibrillation, and the precisely regular "hum" of 60-cycle artifact. The remedy is to have the patient relax, but people who are very sick, especially if they are cold, disoriented, in pain, frightened, or have Parkinson's disease, cannot always do that. A moderate degree of muscle tremor rarely interferes with interpretation. In the case of infants, it may be helpful for someone to hold the patient, with skin contact prevented by a blanket if necessary, while the tracing is recorded.

60-cycle AC interference produces perfectly regular deflections at a rate of 60/s (Fig. 6-2C), and is usually distinguished easily from muscle tremor *(see above)*. It may be of any amplitude in any lead, and may or may not interfere materially with interpretation. It can be eliminated almost always, or at least reduced to insignificance, by removing the source or grounding it to the EKG machine *(see above)*. Techniques for *common mode rejection* found in today's EKG machines have very nearly eliminated this problem.

Wandering of the baseline up and down is the result of motion of an electrode with relation to the skin, and is more common in precordial leads than frontal ones because of the unavoidable motion of the chest with respiration (Fig. 6-2D). The remedy is to see that the electrodes are attached securely but not so tightly as to cause discomfort, and to help the patient relax. A calm, reassuring, unhurried approach by the technician is important. A moderate degree of wandering of the baseline is acceptable, especially if the patient is a small child and/or uncooperative.

Very *abrupt deflections*, often all the way across the chart and occurring in bursts, mean that there is a defective metal-to-metal

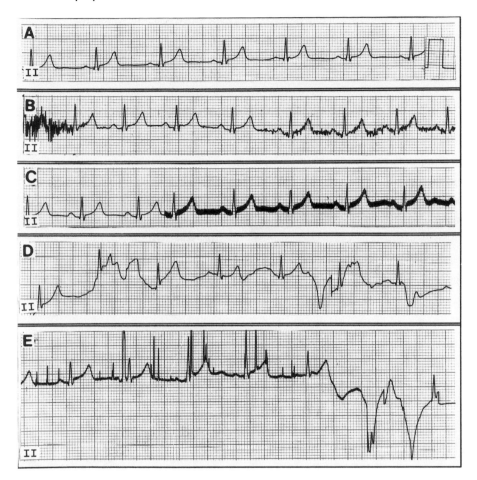

Fig. 6-2. Common baseline artifacts. **A,** normal; **B,** muscle tremor; **C,** 60-cycle AC interference; **D,** loose electrode-to-skin connector; **E,** defective metal-to-metal contact.

contact in the system (Fig. 6-2E). The most common place to find this is in the connection of a lead wire to an electrode, and tightening the binding screw will correct it.

Paper speed: Before direct-writing EKG equipment was available, time lines were projected on the tracing during recording, but the nature of modern equipment requires that they be inscribed before the paper is put into the machine. This means that the paper must move at exactly 25 mm/s in order for the space between two small lines on the graph to represent 0.04 s. When the paper speed is 50 mm/s, and this is not recognized, the tracing may be interpreted as showing marked bradycardia, and prolongation of PR, QRS, and QT, and this may be interpreted as suggesting drug or electrolyte effect. Inappropriate paper speed can be suspected easily enough if one knows the patient's heart rate, but it cannot be proved from the tracing itself unless it includes 60-cycle artifact, which will look like 30-cycle artifact, or an automatic calibration pulse that lasts 0.20 s (5 mm for paper speed of 25 mm/s). Most machines offer the option of 50 mm/s paper speed, but there is rarely, if ever, an indication for this. As with use of double gain (p. 98), all components of the tracing are affected equally and no benefit accrues, like speaking very slowly for someone who doesn't understand English.

Indistinctness of the baseline, blurred, too light, or of varying width, is usually a result of improper relation between stylus and paper, and is not a problem with digital equipment. The most common means of recording electrocardiograms until very recently was with a heated stylus writing on heat-sensitive paper drawn tightly over a sharp edge. In this system, the stylus describes an arc of a circle but touches the paper only on the line defined by this edge, and must move exactly parallel to the surface of the writing edge, and equal pressure must be applied across the whole chart. A bent stylus, or one that is too hot, can produce fuzziness of the trace, and an error of insertion of the paper, so that it is not stretched tightly over the edge, can do the same thing.

Errors of Labeling, Crossed Leads

Electrodes may be placed incorrectly, strips may be mounted improperly on prelabeled forms, and it is possible with some equipment to plug individual leads into the wrong place in the data acquisition unit of the patient cable. Mistakes are made by even the best of technicians, and, when this happens, the doctor must recognize it. Patterns help, but systematic description of the tracing can expose errors that would be missed by casual inspection.

Medical students, given the hint that there is a technical error and asked to explain it, often say something like "the leads are switched." Asked which leads, the answer will be "the limb leads," an incomplete explanation at best. Asked again, the response may be that lead I and lead II are crossed, a hypothesis that does not make sense at all in terms of recording, but might explain an error of mounting and labeling. Part of the problem is that the word *lead* is used to mean at least two things (p. 243); the tracing itself, and the wire that is a part of the patient cable. In the first sense, a lead can be "crossed" by being mounted in the wrong position, as when single-channel machines are used; in the second, leads (components of the tracing) are "crossed" because leads (components of the patient cable) are misplaced.

If lead wires have been attached to the patient incorrectly, but all three corners of Einthoven's triangle are represented, i.e., one is attached to each arm and one to a leg, the tracing is complete, but the labels on the frontal leads are not correct; V leads are not affected. It can be interpreted, after appropriate corrections have been made (Fig. 6-3), just as a printed page held upside down can be read. If both electrodes of a lead are attached to the legs, though, they represent the same point, the inferior angle of the triangle. There is no difference in potential between them, and a flat line results; the tracing is incomplete, but still contains useful information, and modification of the V leads is imperceptible. Remember that the connection from the patient cable to the right leg is for establishing electrical continuity between the body and the chassis of the EKG machine, grounding (p. 99); it will work no matter where it is placed, but is not part of a lead.

When an error of lead labeling, however brought about, is suspected, a good starting point for identifying it is to recognize that lead aVR almost always looks like aVR; i.e., both P and QRS are almost always negative, and T usually is also. If the lead labeled aVF in a three-channel tracing looks like aVR, for instance, the chances are that the tracing was made with right arm and left leg leads transposed. Misplacement of "limb leads" is almost always reciprocal, but may be clockwise, counterclockwise, or random. The nearly stable feature in precordial leads that can have similar

Lead	Correct connections	Arm leads crossed R↔L	Left leads crossed L↔F	Right leads crossed R↔F	Arm and leg leads crossed ipsilaterally R↔F L↔F	
I	+L −R	+R −L	+F −R	+L −F	+F −F	
II	+F −R	+F −L	+L −R	+F −F	+L −F	
III	+F −L	+F −R	+L −F	+F −L	+L −F	
aVR	+R −(L+F)	+L −(R+F)	+R −(F+L)	+F −(L+F)	+F −(F+L)	
aVL	+L −(R+F)	+R −(L+F)	+F −(R+L)	+L −(F+F)	+F −(F+L)	
aVF	+F −(R+L)	+F −(L+R)	+L −(R+F)	+F −(F+L)	+L −(F+F)	

Fig. 6-3. Schema for identifying crossed leads. The right leg electrode is for grounding, and is equally effective wherever it is attached; it is not a component of any lead. As long as all three corners of the triangle are represented, V leads are not affected. R (and RA) stand for right arm; L (and LA) stand for left arm; and F for the inferior angle of Einthoven's triangle, the symphysis pubis. The left leg (LL) is usually used for F, but the right one (RL) will work as well. When an error of frontal lead placement is suspected, identify the probable mistake in the empty column, and test its validity by substituting in the formulae in the first column. The four most common examples of this problem are demonstrated.

value is the terminal negativity of P in V1. If V1 and V3 are transposed, for instance, or precordial leads are recorded, or mounted, in reverse order, recognition of this tiny finding can prevent an erroneous diagnosis of an infarct.

The application of Einthoven's triangle illustrated in Fig. 6-3 is a convenient method of testing proposed explanations for these errors, and the following list of the usual patterns of this group of artifacts can help.

Complexes in Lead I are "Upside Down"

The arm leads are crossed; the left arm lead is on the right arm, and vice versa. When this happens, the polarity of lead I is reversed, the lead labeled II is really III, III is really II, and aVR and aVL are swapped; aVF and the V leads are not changed. All the information is present, it simply needs to be viewed differently; correction is easy. If the QRS is perpendicular to lead I (+90° or –90°), recognition that the arm leads are crossed depends on orientation of P, and if there is atrial fibrillation, i.e., no P, it may not be possible, but in these circumstances it makes little difference.

An alternative to be considered when arm leads are suspected of being crossed is that the heart is crossed. Dextrocardia produces exactly the same picture in frontal leads as that due to crossed arm leads, but a very different one in precordial leads. Crossing the arm leads does not make any difference in the V leads, all three corners of the triangle are still represented in the central terminal (p. 88), but when there is dextrocardia the lead labeled V1 has the position relative to the heart that V2 normally does, and vice versa, complexes grow smaller and more negative farther to the left, and V6 corresponds to V6R in the normal heart.

Lead I is Flat

Arm leads are on the legs, and leg leads are on the arms. Remember that there are only three corners in a triangle; the connection to the right leg is for grounding and does not relate to the tracing otherwise. A ground can be provided from any position on the body; the right leg just happens to be the one used. When arm and leg leads are swapped ipsilaterally, lead I is flat because both electrodes involved are attached to the same angle of the triangle, the symphysis pubis, and there is no difference between a point; Einthoven's premises leave room for a tiny blip corresponding to QRS, but often there is no deflection at all. The leads labeled II and III are both III, but upside down. Only two angles of the triangle are represented, and the tracing, though not useless, is incomplete. V leads are changed very little.

Lead II is Flat

Right arm and leg leads are crossed. The trace in lead II is flat because both its electrodes are attached to legs, to the same point on the volume conductor, and there is no difference in potential between them. The lead labeled I is III upside down, lead III is valid, and the tracing is incomplete. If P, QRS, and T were all directed to −30° or +150°, the picture would be similar, but this is not likely to occur. When there is atrial fibrillation, or atrial activity is not clear, and T voltage is low, the picture may be hard to distinguish from this artifact. Modification of the V leads is not detectable.

Lead III is Flat

Left arm and right leg leads are crossed. Lead I becomes lead II, lead II is unchanged, and lead III is missing. The tracing is incomplete; but the V leads are hardly affected.

Lead aVR, aVL, or aVF is Flat

A lead wire from the patient cable is defective. Though not uselss, the tracing is incomplete.

Miscellaneous Artifacts

When a Q wave in lead III raises the question of an *inferior infarct in a patient thought not to have had one,* or if the pattern suggests an infarct but "just doesn't look right," the possibility that the tracing was recorded with the *left arm lead on the left leg and the left leg lead on the left arm* must be considered. When this happens, the lead labeled II is really I, I is II, and III is upside down. This is a two-edged problem; it may either simulate an infarct when there is not one, or obscure it when there is. With only one tracing, it can only be suspected; if a previous one is available for comparison, it can be recognized easily, but it still may not be clear which of the two was made with the left leads crossed. It will help to remember that transposition of the connections of a lead reverses the polarity of all components, not just QRS. Lead III is often a transitional lead; most forces generated during both depolarization and repolarization are nearly perpendicular to it, and tiny change in their direction can make the difference between positive and negative in their projection on it while not being noticeable in leads to which they are more nearly parallel. If the complexes are small, especially if there is atrial fibrillation and low T voltage, there may be very little deflection at all in Lead III, even when connections are normal.

A precordial lead may be swapped with an extremity lead, and chest leads may be recorded in reverse order or from the right side of the chest, or mixed in any combination; transposition of V1 and V3, for instance, is especially common and produces a pattern of anterior infarction that can be very convincing. Terminal negativity of P in the lead labeled V3 is a strong hint that this has occurred.

Other possibilities for producing artifacts are numerous, and some are not nearly so easy to recognize as those of recording; even hiccups can simulate P waves, for instance;[779] every new method introduces new opportunities for error,[865–869] and it is a good rule that, when one artifact is detected, others should be suspected.

Miscellaneous Methods
Related to Electrocardiography

Telemetry

Telemetry means measurement from a distance; display of tracings at the central station in an ordinary monitoring unit is an example. The idea is not new; Einthoven wrote about it in 1906.[688] Electrocardiograms have been transmitted from the moon, and monitoring of ambulatory patients in the hospital is routine. Another example is transmission of electrocardiograms by telephone, either directly or by facsimile, for interpretation by a consultant at a distance, and this has been a practical option since 1953.[931]

Ambulatory (Holter) Monitoring

There are two clinical problems, chest pain and arrhythmias, in which evidence available only by electrocardiography is of great value, but which are intermittent. Continuous recording of the electrocardiogram over a period of hours is helpful in these situations and can be accomplished by means of a small, battery-powered recorder that the patient carries while continuing regular activities, i.e., is ambulatory. It is often called by the name of its inventor, Holter.[780] This technique can be used to document transient ST displacement as with coronary insufficiency, but its most important application is for detection of disorders of impulse formation and conduction, arrhythmias; when coronary insufficiency is suspected, the patient can be studied more efficiently in the laboratory (p. 219). Information is recorded and played back rapidly through a device that analyzes it and permits writing selected segments in real time.[386,610,685] Artifacts may be a problem here as in all other aspects of electrocardiography.[611,679]

Lead III in Deep Inspiration

A strip of lead III made during deep inspiration has been used from time to time to help in evaluation of Q3, and sometimes to accentuate disorders of cardiac mechanism,[394,489,496,532] but adds very little.

Esophageal Leads

Leads have been made from the esophagus for special purposes, such as identification of P waves when they are not clear from the surface tracing, since the very early days of electrocardiography, and are still utilized occasionally, most recently in an effort to record a better signal from the atrium for definition of P for computer recognition.[782,783,789]

Facsimile

Once a tracing has been recorded, labeled, and identified, it must be made available to the doctor who is going to interpret it. If the interpreter is at a distance, there are electronic means for transmitting it and receiving the report. The most adaptable, inexpensive, and useful of these is facsimile. The word means likeness, or copy; pictures in today's local newspaper showing events that happened thousands of miles away this morning are facsimiles, and so are ordinary photocopies. Devices for sending and receiving facsimile by telephone are almost ubiquitous now, inexpensive, and can be used with any modular telephone. An electrocardiogram made on any machine at any time can be transmitted easily, a report can be returned to the local site, and the primary doctor, or nurse in the CCU, can discuss the problem with the consultant while each has a copy of the tracing. This system can be used efficiently and effectively in combination with computer analysis (p. 224).

SEVEN

Analytic Methods

The purpose of this brief chapter is to call attention to the similarity between physical examination and analysis of an electrocardiogram: vital signs, inspection, palpation, percussion, and auscultation in the one, and rates and intervals, orientation, duration, amplitude, and contour in the other, four functions in each case, as basic as addition, subtraction, multiplication, and division in mathematics.

Examination of a Series of Beats

Rates and intervals document the relation of atria to ventricles in a series of beats, as well as the duration of events within a beat, and, like temperature, pulse, respiration, and blood pressure of the physical examination, can be determined objectively and quantitatively and are recorded first.

Rates

It is probably safe to assume that everybody understands *rate* to refer to events-per-time, in this case beats-per-minute. Most of the time, *heart* rate really means ventricular rate, and this is acceptable because it is understood universally. Atrial rate and ventricular rate are not always the same, however, and the admonition (p. 6) to be as specific as possible can be applied in thinking, even if not always in speaking and writing. One of the major reasons to make an EKG is to display the relation between atrial and ventricular activity, especially when some "arrhythmia," some disorder of impulse formation and/or conduction, is suspected.

Rhythm

The word *rhythm* is a barrier of sorts to understanding and accurate reporting of findings in a tracing. It is a common word in everyone's vocabulary, referring to timing of events in a series, basically regular or irregular, sometimes in patterns, syncopated, three-quarter time, or iambic pentameter. It retains this meaning in electrocardiography, but, in addition, is used to designate the origin(s) and distribution of impulses in the heart, events that have been known since the earliest days of the discipline as the "mechanism of the heartbeat," or just "the mechanism." The rhythm of these events is an important descriptor, and those in the upper heart must be considered separately from those in the lower, but it would be clumsy to talk about the rhythm of the rhythm, and nobody does. The result is such illogical statements as "regular rate and rhythm." Rate is great or small and is expressed quantitatively in beats per minute; cardiac rhythm is basically regular or irregular, and "cardiac" in this sense really means ventricular. Atrial rhythm is rarely noted.

Intervals

Interval means the same thing in electrocardiography as elsewhere, the distance between two points; in the EKG, points in time. It is interesting that, of the three intervals, PR, QRS, and QT, two refer to the duration of inevitably related processes within a beat, whereas the other describes the relation between independent systems. Another interval is the cycle length, the time from a point in one beat to the same point in the next. This is not measured, or identified as an interval, but is handled as rate (short cycle length, fast rate; long, slow) and rhythm (constant, regular; inconstant, irregular).

The duration of all intervals (and waves) varies inversely with rate, and is measured in the lead in which it is longest *and* can be determined with the most confidence—two observations that sometimes are not clear in the same lead, forcing a small choice. In each case, the B point is a given, and only one other point remains to be determined. The temptation is to call intervals too close; it is important to recognize the limits of the method and the range of normal for each measurement—as well as the consequences of estimating them wrong.

Examination of a Single Beat

The unknown being evaluated in electrocardiography is energy. The idea of energy is probably understood by everybody, and so is the law of the conservation of energy, that it changes form but is not destroyed. Quantitative discussion of it in terms that most of us can comprehend, however, is something else, and can get complicated. The energy manifest in the tracing was stored only a moment ago as protein, carbohydrate, and fat, and is in the process of being converted to heat and motion. During the time it writes tracing, though, it is electricity, generated and dissipated within the anatomic and physiologic framework of the heart. Electricity, like gravity, has characteristics that have been found by experience to be predictable and that can be indicated by words and symbols, making it possible for us to use it without really understanding it.

The EKG machine charts the course through time and space of a single point, A, that represents the net result of these events in the heart. As this point moves, its projection on a system of coordinates, whose spatial relation to each other is known, produces a group of curves that provide three-dimensional information. The fixed reference point for these events (Einthoven's single dipole, Wilson's central terminal of zero potential, point B) is the center of the chest at the level of the fourth intercostal space anteriorly. It is represented in the trace by the beginning point of QRS and, for a series of beats, by the baseline (p. 9). Analysis of the orientation, duration, and amplitude of these curves, and the collective expression of these variables as contour, can give information about the anatomy and physiology of the heart not available in any other way.

Orientation

The word *orientation* is based on *orient*, or east, and refers to the alignment of something in space, "the three-dimensional realm in which all material objects are located and in which all events occur"; the three dimensions (or coordinates, or axes) are called left and right, up and down, and front and back, or X, Y, and Z. These facts are well known, and are pointed out here simply because it is so easy to lose sight of their relevance in electrocardiography. The space with which we are concerned is that within the thorax and abdomen, and the three dimensions are indicated as Leads I, aVF, and V1. Each is effectively perpendicular to the other two (p. 89), and so is each of the three planes they define: frontal (XY), horizontal (XZ), and sagittal (YZ). Three mutually orthogonal axes define space in the human body no less than in a room or the cosmos (*see* Fig. 2-3.)

Everyone knows this and is aware of it when speaking of hearts and lungs, hands and feet, tables and chairs, but it is less obvious in something as symbolic as an electrocardiogram. Orientation of the parts of the tracing has always been central to analysis but is called by so many names that the feature itself, direction in space, is not always recognizable, e.g., axis for the frontal QRS and transition for the horizontal, elevation and depression for ST, and positive and negative, upright and inverted, for any wave or deflection.

The symbol, however, the tracing, is not abstract but a collection of lines, graphs, XY plots with recurrent waveforms that have names and can be defined in millimeters, milliseconds, degrees, and contours. Instructions for determining the orientation of each element are given in Chapter Two.

Duration

The duration of a wave or an interval is the time from its beginning to its end, and the most difficult part of choosing a figure for it is to recognize the limits of the method. If the limits are exceeded, if the numbers are called too close, or if it is assumed that a computer readout to the third decimal place is necessarily significant, the patient may suffer.

Amplitude

The amplitude of waves and deflections, their "magnitude" in vector terminology, is discussed in all texts but, as with orientation, so many names and measures for it are used (elevation and depression, displacement, marked and slight, low, tall, great, small, and voltage, millimeters, and millivolts) that the value itself, the distance of a moving point from a fixed one, manifest as the position of the trace above or below the baseline, is not always recognizable. To realize what is being identified, and name it, reduces the number of variables to be dealt with and simplifies the process of describing and interpreting a tracing.

Contour

The shape of a wave or segment in a given lead, its contour or configuration, represents the projection on that lead of a series of events that can be expressed as points, or instantaneous vectors (p. 70), and the rate of change of the orientation and amplitude of these varies. Orientation and amplitude can be reduced to numbers, but the product of their interaction during the time it takes to generate a wave or segment can be described only by adjectives; real and important as it is, contour, like truth and beauty, is in the eye of the beholder. The subject has received little attention, and there is almost no refuge to be had in jargon, no escape from saying what one means, using everyday words, and this is not bad. Students facing the challenge of describing EKG contours for the first time often repeat information already noted quantitatively (the QRS is described as wide, for instance, or tall) and this adds nothing. If the contour is not abnormal, then it must be described as normal, but this does not add anything either unless everybody knows just what it excludes. An adjective works only if the alternatives are known, a very big if that carries with it a considerable chance for error. The limits of the method, and the doctor's responsibility for doing the right thing, are big factors.

The features that can be quantified—rates, intervals, orientation, duration, and amplitude—will have been described by the time contour (of P, QRS, ST, and T) must be handled. Normal contours, and departures from normal, of individual waves and segments are discussed in Chapter Two as they are encountered in describing the tracing.

Interpretation

Findings on physical examination are coordinated with those from history and laboratory study to produce a diagnosis with three components—topography, etiology, and manifestations—and those from the EKG lead to an interpretation that also has three components—mechanism, structure, and function. An EKG is a laboratory study, and whatever information it contains must be converted to language that makes it as directly relevant to signs and symptoms as possible.

EIGHT

Disorders of Impulse Formation

This chapter and the next are concerned with "arrhythmias," abnormalities of impulse formation and conduction. The methods introduced in Chapter Two, and described in detail in Chapter Seven, will be used to point out the features in the tracing that identify as nearly as possible the location of the pacemaker for the atria, that for the ventricles, the rate and rhythm of each, and the causal relation between them, or its absence. The means by which any abnormalities thus identified were brought about and sustained will be considered separately, and the dilemma of how to choose precise and mutually exclusive names for them will be discussed. Explanations are critical because they are the basis for management, but they should follow statement of the problem, not replace it, and some of the names in common use imply explanations without having said what is being explained. *Why* abnormalities occur is teleology, and not the subject at hand.

Background

Important discoveries in cardiac anatomy, physiology, and pathology were made during the same years that electrocardiography was developing, each contributing to the others; it was the time of Wenckebach, Mayer, His and Tawara, of Keith and Flack, Lewis, Mines, and Garrey, of Mobitz, Starling, and Herrick. By the mid-1920s the function of the heart as a pump had been studied extensively, and most of the anatomic and physiologic principles governing impulse formation and conduction that underlie current thinking were known. Waller's demonstration in 1887 (p. 66), that electrical activity precedes muscle contraction, had presaged the first, and for a long time almost the only, clinical role of electrocardiography, and display of the electrical events that control the pump is still perhaps its most critical application; much of the information needed for diagnosis and management of problems in this area can be had by no other means.

Evolution of the discipline of clinical electrophysiology as a subspecialty within cardiology has produced not only a broad range of new possibilities for patient care, but also, as all specialties do, a language of its own, in this case, a jargon that has much in common with that of traditional electrocardiography but is not quite the same, limiting to some extent the transfer of new knowledge to the surface tracing and the patient. Specialized meanings are ascribed to everyday words (rhythm, ectopic), there is redundancy (ectopic atrial), different names are used for the same phenomenon (reentry, reciprocal, echo, circus), combinations of findings are treated as if they were indivisible (flutter, fibrillation, SVT, wide complex tachycardia), there are nebulous concepts (incessant), and individual findings are not identified as specifically as possible (heart block). Even "bradycardia" and "tachycardia" are confusing; "brady" and "tachy" mean slow and fast, but rate can be specified quantitatively, and "cardia" doesn't distinguish between atria and ventricles. The word "arrhythmia" itself is anomalous, implying irregularity of rhythm, but some "arrhythmias" are perfectly regular.

Survey of Anatomic, Physiologic, Semantic, and Instrumental Features Relevant at This Point

Cells in the heart can be classified in two groups according to their primary function, those that generate and transmit electrical signals, and those that contract in response to the signals; Mackenzie called them genetic and muscular.[917] The electrically active ones can be subdivided into those that have the intrinsic property of initiating impulses, automaticity, found in clusters in the sinus node and AV junction, and scattered in atria and ventricles, and those better suited for transmission. Our chief concern now is with the first group, including the second only to the extent that it relates to continuation of ectopic activity. Abnormalities of conduction between the origin of an impulse and its target contractile elements, AV and IV block, will be discussed in Chapters Nine and Ten.

There are two potentially independent electrical systems in the heart, one in the atria and one in the ventricles, and the fastest pacemaker available to each controls its rate. In the normal state, impulses arise spontaneously in the sinus node, spread rapidly over the atria, very slowly through the AV junction, and thence almost instantaneously to the ventricles (p. 75). These characteristics describe a kind of an electrical funnel with the atria as collecting chamber and the AV junction as spout. The His–Purkinje system represents the open space between the funnel and the container into which it empties, and the ventricles represent the container. The output of the funnel is a function of both the rate of input and the flow permitted by its narrowest part, and can be modified by change in either or both.

Before the origin of an impulse can be identified, certain limitations must be recognized. Signals generated outside the heart are usually easy to differentiate from those from arising within it (p. 102), and potentials produced by atrial repolarization are too small to influence the surface tracing, but there are still three to be reckoned with, atrial and ventricular depolarization and ventricular repolarization. Ventricular depolarization and repolarization are necessarily sequential, but the atria may depolarize at any time without regard to events in the ventricles, and the trace reflects the position of a *single point*, representing the net of *all* of these. Distinguishing atrial from ventricular activity in the EKG is kind of like making sense of the messages from two radio stations broadcasting on the same frequency; there are two signals but only one transducer. The AV diagram, or Engelmann laddergram, shown in Fig. 8-1 can be very helpful in unraveling their true identities and interrelations.

Whatever help there is to be had from the tracing depends on translation into terms that relate its meaning to anatomy and physiology, signs and symptoms, and use of common words to mean something different from what they do in everyday life is a stumbling block in this process. One that figures prominently in the classification that follows is *ectopic*, an adjective that means "outside the normal place;" impulse formation at any place other than the sinus node is ectopic, abnormal by definition, but ranging in impor-

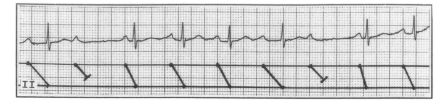

Fig. 8-1. Engelmann's laddergram, or AV diagram, a method of analysis older than electrocardiography itself. It helps in separation of atrial activity from ventricular, and much more complex forms than this one can be devised.[698]

tance from insignificant to life threatening. Impulses that arise outside the sinus node but proximal to the bifurcation of the Bundle of His are *supraventricular*; distal to that point, *ventricular*. Those with rates slower than sinus, appearing when the sinus node fails to fire, or impulses from it, or from some other faster focus, are kept from reaching the ventricles, represent escape of the slower focus as a defense measure, functioning by *default*; those with rates greater than sinus, taking over pacemaker function aggressively, are described as *usurping*. The common ectopic mechanisms will be considered under these traditional and useful headings, objectively demonstrable features first, and the subjective process of explanation and labeling later. It is easier to set up an organized approach than to make the subject matter conform to it, though, and these subdivisions are not always mutually exclusive. Current terminology will prevail in clinical practice, and will be used here, but awareness of its derivation and limitations can aid in its proper use.

No Identifiable Atrial Activity

If the trace is flat between the U wave of one beat and the QRS of the next, it may mean that there is:

1. A midjunctional pacemaker with the atria depolarized at the same time as the ventricles so that P waves simply cannot be seen;

2. Sino-ventricular conduction with the impulse reaching the AV node by way of internodal pathways without depolarizing the atria;[491]
3. Sinus arrest with atrial standstill (and junctional escape);[709,710,889]
4. That atrial complexes are just too small to see [485,498,519] or are oriented perpendicular to the lead; P waves are often very small in elderly people.

Sinus Mechanism and Its Variants

The normal heartbeat is initiated by an impulse that arises in the sinus node, spreads over the atria, producing the P wave, passes through the slowly conducting AV node during the PR interval, and reaches the ventricles, producing the QRS, T, and U. This sequence of events, a one-to-one relation between atria and ventricles with P directed caudad, is called a sinus mechanism. Precisely what rates are to be regarded as fast or slow, "tachy" or "brady," are arbitrary, but some pivotal figures are useful to know. In the adult at rest, the sinus rate is usually between fifty and 100 beats/min, not often below forty, and rarely above 140 except when there is increase in the need for oxygen and/or lessening of its supply, e.g., hyperpyrexia, thyrotoxicosis, shock, acute blood loss, or, most commonly, impairment of oxygen transfer as with lung disease. It is rare for untreated usurping ectopy to occur at a rate slower than 160, but it is not always possible to tell whether a P is of sinus origin or atrial, and at ventricular rates between 140 and 160 there may be doubt. A sinus origin is more common than atrial in this range except when there is flutter with atrial rate of the order of 300 (p. 129). Sinus rhythm is slightly irregular, slower on inhalation and faster on exhalation, especially in youth and old age, *sinus arrhythmia*. If the sinus rate slows abruptly, but not long enough for a lower pacemaker to escape, there is a longer interval than usual between two beats of sinus origin, a *sinus pause*;[745] if the pause is long enough, a junctional pacemaker will *escape* and drive the ventricles (p. 125).

Sinoatrial (SA) Block

Sometimes a single complete cardiac cycle, a PQRST, is missing, although the regular rhythm continues. This is called sinoatrial (SA) block,[67,68,420,421,494,506] the implication being that an impulse was formed in the sinus node but did not enter the atria. The terminology of SA block is exceedingly complex and inconstant, and the hypotheses and assumptions that underlie the concept are even more obscure than in most disorders of mechanism. Its clinical importance is hard to evaluate, ranging from insignificant to catastrophic when it is complete and no lower pacemaker takes over, literally cardiac standstill.[420,421,651] In some instances it may be provoked, or abolished, by quinidine.[651]

Wandering Atrial Pacemaker

The implication of "wandering atrial pacemaker"[36,504] is that some beats arise in the sinus node, some from sites in the atria, and some from the AV junction. It is recognized by P waves whose configurations vary within a given lead and whose PR intervals shorten as the pacemaker approaches the AV junction. The term is used loosely, though, and often seems to mean simply that there are PACs, or that the pacemaker alternates between sinus node and AV junction. It is not likely to be important and can be thought of as a variant of normal.

The *sick sinus syndrome* is a spectrum of clinical problems, chiefly weakness and syncope, resulting from instability of the sinus node. The heart rate varies between very slow and very fast, sometimes including periods of asystole and of atrial tachycardia; it has been called *sluggish sinus* and *brady–tachy* syndrome also. The EKG picture depends upon documentation in a series of tracings; the diagnosis is not made from a single tracing.[521,533,536,652,654,745]

Atrial Dissociation, or *interatrial block*, implies that the atria function separately, producing two P waves, one from the left atrium and one from the right. It is a rare phenomenon, and details of definitions vary.[74,84,424,476,479,524,892]

Intraatrial block, evidence of delay in conduction through the atria, is defined even less clearly in the literature and is recognized by widening and notching of P.[74,492,577] It may represent atrial disease, but is not well understood.

Default Mechanisms of Supraventricular Origin

Impulses that arise anywhere above the bifurcation of the His Bundle, whether in the sinus node, an atrium, or the AV junction, are distributed to the ventricles over the same pathways and give rise to the same QRS-T pattern. Their origin is identified by the atrial complexes they produce, and, except when there is atrial fibrillation, this means P waves, especially their orientation and whether they precede or follow QRS. Instructions for analysis of atrial activity are found on p. 19. Possibilities are considered below. The difference between default and usurpation is an important concept, but distinction between them is not based entirely on the rate or location of the ectopic focus; the presence or absence of a sinus mechanism or atrial fibrillation in the same tracing is a factor also (p. 133).

Default Mechanisms of Atrial Origin

When the sinus node fails to fire, the next fastest pacemaker escapes and paces the heart at a regular rhythm. If this is in an atrium, and if the terminology were consistent, it would be called atrial bradycardia, but this term is encountered rarely. If it is in the cephalic part of an atrium, it may produce P waves that are indistinguishable from those of sinus origin; in the midsection, Ps that are not identifiable with confidence, if at all; and if it is in the caudal portion, it produces retrograde Ps and is called low atrial, or high junctional *(see below)*. The pattern produced by an artificial pacemaker depends on the position of the pacing electrode.

Default Mechanisms of Junctional Origin (Fig. 8-2)

These mechanisms occur when the sinus node fails to fire, or when there is third degree AV block, and they are characterized by regular QRS rhythm at a rate slower than would be expected from the sinus node. If P waves are visible at all, there is one for each

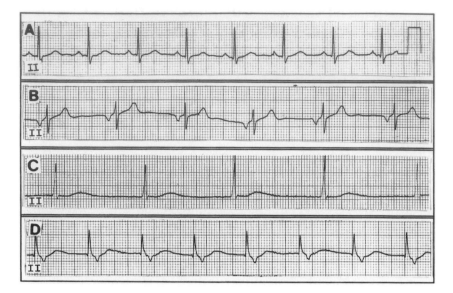

Fig. 8-2. Supraventricular default mechanisms. **(A)** is sinus for control; **(B)** high junctional (or low atrial); **(C)** midjunctional (or nodal); and **(D)** low junctional (or His Bundle).

QRS, they are negative in Leads II, III, and aVF, and often prominent and conspicuously V-shaped. QRS is narrow unless there is a defect of intraventricular conduction. These have been called *nodal* mechanisms, and sometimes still are,[706] but this is probably not accurate, since there is evidence that the AV node itself does not initiate impulses.[85] The term has been replaced for practical purposes by *junctional*, designating an ill-defined area from low in the atria to the bifurcation of the Bundle of His.[97–99,487,557] It has been the custom for a long time to identify these as upper junctional (or coronary sinus or low atrial) in origin when the retrograde P precedes QRS, lower when it follows, and midjunctional if no atrial activity is visible,[57,73,86,87–96,455] but the clinical value of this is dubious; any of them is seen as a normal expression of intrinsic automaticity released by the absence of a faster pacemaker. Contour and timing of P and QRS in these mechanisms are influenced by varying degrees of antegrade and retrograde conduction delay, and may not be explicable on the basis of anatomy alone.

Usurping Mechanisms of Supraventricular Origin: Supraventricular Tachycardias

Any mechanism arising above the bifurcation of the Bundle of His, whatever its rate and rhythm, is of supraventricular origin, and "tachycardia" simply means fast heart. Taken literally, "supraventricular tachycardia" is a generic term that does not distinguish among mechanisms of sinus, atrial, or junctional origin, but in practice it implies a junctional focus and, to some extent, a clinical picture *(see below)*. Usurping mechanisms originating in the atria are given names (atrial tachycardia, flutter, and fibrillation), that describe them individually.

Continued firing of an ectopic focus presents a problem with two parts; how the abnormal activity was initiated, and how it is sustained. If a tracing shows the first ectopic beat, some information about how it was initiated may be inferred, and this may be useful in planning prophylaxis, but when abnormal activity is already in progress the immediate question is not how to prevent another episode but how to stop this one. A premise regarding the means by which activity is sustained is the basis for management of the patient, but before this can be considered, the problem must be identified, named, and this requires analysis and interpretation.

The rate and rhythm of atria and ventricles can be determined easily in most instances, but the anatomic locus of the electrophysiologic lesion, and the cause-and-effect relation between atrial and ventricular activity, when there is one, must be deduced from the intrinsic characteristics of atrial and ventricular complexes and their timing. In the pages that follow, the common arrhythmias are taken up in the order of increasing atrial rate, labeling each feature of the tracing as objectively as possible, distinguishing between description and interpretation. The subject is discussed in all EKG books, and no two say exactly the same thing. Critical reading of other texts is encouraged.

Premature Atrial Contractions (PACs)

PACs are the most common form of ectopy, and their name describes them. The P wave of a PAC is premature, and its orientation and contour are different from normal (Fig. 8-3). Those that originate near the cephalic end of an atrium may be indistinguish-

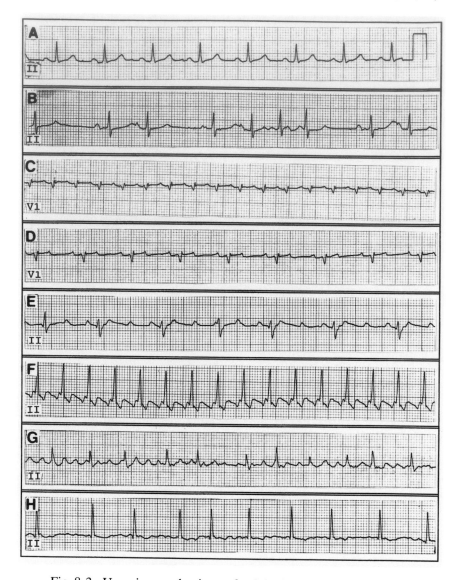

Fig. 8-3. Usurping mechanisms of atrial origin. **(A)** is sinus for control; **(B)** premature atrial contractions (PACs); **(C)** atrial tachycardia, rate 160; **(D)** atrial tachycardia with block, 160/180 (the same patient as B); **(E)** another example of atrial tachycardia with block, atrial rate 190, varying second degree AV block, ventricular rate about 70; **(F)** classic atrial flutter, 300/150; **(G)** coarse atrial fibrillation, or *flutter-fibrillation*; and **(H)** fine atrial fibrillation.

able from sinus beats, the origin of those from midatrial sites may be mostly inferential, and those arising near the caudal end are negative in leads II, III, and aVF, reflecting retrograde depolarization of the atria. The PR interval of a PAC may be shorter than normal, or longer, depending on its timing and the refractory periods of the tissues involved;[423] if it occurs early enough, it may be *blocked* completely,[76] producing an early, ectopic P not followed by a QRS. The QRS-T of most PACs is almost exactly the same as that of sinus beats in the same lead, but small differences are common and large ones can occur (*see ventricular aberration*, p. 169). The pause following the PAC may or may not be compensatory, i.e., the interval between the preceding and following beats may or may not be the same as if it had not occurred. PACs may be frequent or rare, unifocal or multifocal in origin, isolated or in groups. If one follows each sinus beat, there is bigeminy due to PACs, or *atrial bigeminy*; when several occur consecutively, they are often called a *salvo* (*see multifocal atrial tachycardia*, p. 133).

Atrial Tachycardia

Usurping supraventricular ectopy, defined as a clinical entity, is common, usually benign, and characteristically episodic, with abrupt onset and offset, rate between 160–220, regular rhythm, lasting from a few beats to a few hours, and often seen in young people with no other evidence of heart disease. This has been known for a long time as *paroxysmal atrial tachycardia*, or *PAT*, but the EKG picture implied by this name, P waves of ectopic origin, each followed by a QRS that is not wide unless there is an associated IV conduction defect, is rare, especially in adults. It does occur in children, however, and, if persistent instead of paroxysmal, may result in congestive failure. Atrial tachycardia is almost always associated with second degree AV block (p. 152). The clinical syndrome indicated above is usually called just *supraventricular tachycardia*, or SVT (p. 133).

Atrial Tachycardia with Block, and Atrial Flutter

Normal AV junctional tissue can conduct no more than about 180–200 impulses per minute,[921] and when more than this reach it not all of them can be transmitted to the ventricles, i.e., there is second degree AV block. It is interesting that, with sinus rates in this range, there is no AV block, and this is probably explained by enhancement of AV conduction by catecholamines when the mechanism is of sinus origin but not when it is ectopic (p. 154). At rates greater than about 300–340, atrial activity is no longer organized and predictable (p. 131). Usurping atrial ectopy at rates greater than the normal AV junction can conduct occurs in two forms, *atrial tachycardia with block* and *atrial flutter*.

When the atrial rate is between about 180–220, and P waves are discrete and not negative in II, III, and aVF, the combination is known traditionally as *PAT with block* (Fig. 8-3). The tracing shows only the mechanism, though, not its paroxysmal nature, and this is being recognized increasingly by calling it only *atrial tachycardia with block*, including numbers for atrial and ventricular rates: "atrial tachycardia with block, 180/70." P waves are likely to be very small. It is possible, of course, for there to be impairment of AV conduction at the same time that input from the atria is abnormally rapid, and digitalis excess may explain both.[80,82,922]

The other form is called *atrial flutter*. The tracing typically shows continuous, regular oscillation of the trace, producing a serrated, "sawtooth," or "picket fence" pattern in Leads II, III, and aVF, a useful description, but one that, taken literally, precludes even definition of a P, much less calling it positive or negative. In most instances, however, supported by evidence in other leads, commonly V1, P waves can be separated from each other, and are negative in II, III, and aVF (Fig. 8-3). The atrial rate is often very nearly exactly 300, ventricular 150, but rates vary widely and the P:QRS ratio need not be fixed.

It is helpful to remember that atrial and ventricular activity may be in progress at the same time; otherwise, a P merged with the initial part of QRS may be seen as an R or a Q, depending on its sign, or as an R or an S when continuous with the distal end. A P superimposed on ST can be mistaken for the T wave, but the improbably brief QT implified by this interpretation would point to the error. A P that occurs at the same time as QRS may not be identifiable. The importance of a firm concept of the baseline (p. 9) cannot be overemphasized.

The critical findings in both atrial tachycardia with block and flutter are P waves of ectopic origin and at a rapid rate, some of which are not conducted to the ventricles. Different P rates and morphologies probably reflect different locations of the electrophysiologic lesion and the means by which activity is sustained (*see* p. 137), but the abnormality in both is confined to the atria.

"Atrial tachycardia with block" is easy to accept as a complete and objective statement of the findings in a tracing; it identifies each of separate components, and does not include an explanation for either. The means by which ectopic impulse formation is sustained is not clear, probably local automaticity at a point relatively high in an atrium, either rapid phase four depolarization or a local circus. In this setting, AV block is evidence of normal AV function. In the case of flutter, though, both findings are covered by a single word, and that word has other meanings as well. Not only is it used often to include atrial tachycardia with block as described above, but also as the name for a clinical entity, and, in the present state of things, to imply intraatrial reentry (p. 138) as the explanation for both. Confusion can be lessened by limiting the EKG diagnosis of "flutter" to tracings with negative Ps in II, III, and aVF.

The expression *1:1 flutter*[77,475,607] is used sometimes to describe a mechanism of atrial origin at a rate above that at which some degree of AV block is usually seen, a picture hard to define as different from atrial tachycardia *(above)* and other forms of SVT or *narrow complex tachycardia (below)*, but meaningful if typical flutter, or atrial tachycardia, has been demonstrated in another tracing.

Atrial Fibrillation

The atria cannot be depolarized in an organized, repetitive manner at rates much above about 300/min in most people, hardly ever 400. Somewhere in this range, coordinated activity deteriorates, and individual fibers, or bundles of fibers, begin to function independently in a random fashion, i.e., to fibrillate (when the word is pronounced with a long "i," it is onomatopoeic). Before electrocardiographic studies clarified what was going on, the clinical condition associated with this had been known by such wonderfully descriptive names as *chaos cordis*, *delirium cordis*, and *pulsus irregularis perpetuum*. When Mackenzie began to correlate the clinical and electrocardiographic findings, he reasoned that the impulses must originate between atria and ventricles, and called it *nodal rhythm*,[917] a name that was soon to take on a different meaning.

When the atria are fibrillating, the AV junction is subjected continuously to impulses at varying rates and strengths, and not all of them reach the ventricles. Second degree AV block is a built-in part of atrial fibrillation, reflecting the normal filtering effect of the AV junction; if this were not present, there would be ventricular fibrillation and the question would be moot. The electrocardiographic diagnosis depends on irregular undulation of the trace between ventricular complexes, "f" waves (Fig. 8-3). These may be coarse and obvious, or so small that they are not clearly identifiable, but in either case the baseline is not exactly the same between any two pairs of contiguous QRSs in the same lead. Irregularity of ventricular rhythm is typical of atrial fibrillation, but not necessary for the diagnosis, and it may be more difficult to recognize in an electrocardiogram than on physical examination, where apical-radial pulse deficit, variation in pulse volume, and intensity of heart sounds helps. When ventricular rate is very rapid or very slow, careful measurement of cycle lengths may be necessary to demonstrate it, and it is possible to have atrial fibrillation with regular ventricular rhythm, as with third degree AV block or acceleration of a junctional pacemaker (p. 133).

Comment

Atrial fibrillation is the only chronic cardiac arrhythmia compatible with health, and may persist for many years without other evidence of heart disease or other electrocardiographic abnormality. It may be familial[596] or idiopathic ("lone"), and it may be asymptomatic. It is rare in infants. The ventricular rate with atrial fibrillation covers the same range as with a sinus mechanism, between about 40 and 200/min. Its two important manifestations are emboli from thrombi in the ineffectively contracting chambers, and lessening of the pumping efficiency of the heart by loss of presystolic injection of blood into the ventricles. It does not by itself produce heart failure, but does contribute by removing the "atrial kick," and is often secondary to lesions that already have overloaded the heart or diminished its pumping effectiveness, mitral valve disease and/or atherosclerosis. Whether treatment is indicated, and, if so, what form it should take, depends on the larger clinical setting. Reversion can almost always be effected by either pharmacologic or electrical means, but atrial fibrillation is a result of disease, not a disease itself, and, unless the underlying problem is corrected, reversion has no lasting effect.

Impure Flutter, or Flutter-Fibrillation

Atrial activity may be repetitive and discrete at a rate of 300 or more in some places, deteriorate into irregularity as the tracing continues, and become organized again later on. To assign a separate name to this has little if any clinical value; it simply serves to emphasize the often arbitrary difference between *flutter* and *fibrillation*. It may be possible to identify P waves in one lead and not in another recorded simultaneously, demonstrating the weakness of including continuous atrial activity as part of the definition of flutter. There are few absolutes in biological systems, and distinction between atrial flutter and atrial fibrillation is not one of them. When the question arises, it is usually more judicious from a clinical point of view to call it fibrillation than flutter.

Unilateral Atrial Fibrillation

Unilateral atrial fibrillation has been reported.[84] *Multifocal atrial tachycardia* occurs when more than one atrial focus is active,[78,79,520] and distinction from atrial fibrillation may be arbitrary.

Tachycardias of Junctional Origin

In all the mechanisms discussed above, the electrophysiologic lesion is in the atria. When ectopic activity is confined to the AV junction, QRS is narrow, as with the atrial mechanisms, but the ventricular rhythm is nearly always perfectly regular, and atrial activity is not always identifiable. These mechanisms are often lumped under such terms as *accelerated junctional mechanisms*, *narrow complex tachycardia*, or, most frequently, *supraventricular tachycardia*, or SVT. Other labels are more explanatory than descriptive, and based on current understanding of the means by which activity is sustained *(see below)*.

Accelerated Junctional Mechanism

Accelerated junctional mechanism is the name applied when, in the presence of sinus activity or atrial fibrillation, and normal AV conduction, narrow QRS complexes occur with a regular rhythm at a rate greater than default but less than typical of usurpation. The ventricles are subject to activation from either of two supraventricular pacemakers, and, when they fail to respond to a sinus impulse because of refractoriness following activation from the junctional focus, there is *AV dissociation* (p. 154). When the rate of the junctional focus is almost exactly the same as sinus, whether because of slowing of sinus or acceleration of junctional, the relation between P and QRS does not vary perceptibly in the time frame of a tracing, there is a P for each QRS, but no causal relation between them, and this is called *isorhythmic dissociation*.[104,371,560,655] *Interference dissociation*[153–155] describes substantially the same situation as *accelerated junctional pacemaker*, but recognizes that some sinus beats are conducted. It has been called a "physiologic arrhythmia."[655]

Acceleration of a mechanism of junctional origin may be evidence of digitalis excess, febrile states, or inflammatory disease, but *acceleration* is not defined quantitatively; rate can be stated in beats per minute. When there is no other atrial activity, a junctional pacemaker is effectively a variant of normal.

Junctional Tachycardia

Junctional tachycardia is a term that is not used very often, but, from an electrocardiographic point of view, would be a logical name for those mechanisms with narrow QRS in which retrograde Ps precede or follow QRS, or atrial activity is not identifiable. When a retrograde P precedes QRS (Fig. 8-4), the traditional interpretation, that it proceeds from a low atrial or *high junctional* focus (the terms are interchangeable), has much to recommend it. This picture is common with rates in the default range but rare with rapid ones, and no clear label for the latter has evolved. The pattern of a QRS of normal duration, regular rhythm, and no identifiable atrial activity suggests a *midjunctional* origin, and this is an acceptable interpretation at default rates, but at usurping ones it is more likely to be called *AV nodal reentrant tachycardia*, both locating the abnormal-

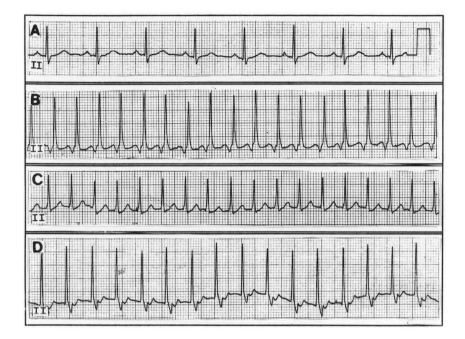

Fig. 8-4. Usurping mechanisms of junctional origin, *supraventricular tachycardia*. (**A**) is sinus for control; (**B**) high junctional, rare; and (**C**) midjunctional, commonly called *AV nodal reentry*. In (**D**) a retrograde P follows QRS, low junctional (or *AV reentry*). Note the similarity between these mechanisms and those in Fig. 8-2.

ity and explaining it. The reasoning is that there is a looping process within the AV junctional area that fires the atria at its upper end and the ventricles at its lower in such rapid sequence that P is written at the same time as QRS and obscured by it.

Whatever name is used, the abnormality in both of these entities is confined to the AV junction. When a retrograde P follows the QRS, though, and is clearly separate from it, current terminology calls it *AV reentrant* tachycardia. The explanation implied by this is that the reentry loop is not confined to the AV junction but involves ventricular tissue and an anomalous peripheral connection between atria and ventricles, e.g., a Kent bundle. Any of these patterns may be clear-cut, but it is common also for a retrograde P to be merged with QRS at either its beginning or its end, making choice among them difficult. Electrophysiologic progress in revealing ever-finer detail has outstripped progress in the nomenclature needed to make it available to nonelectrophysiologists.

Comment

It is usually easy to narrow the choice to one or two of the classifications discussed above, but distinctions blur, and a label that all can agree is appropriate is not always possible. An accurate statement of the findings, recognizing the limitations of the method, would identify a supraventricular mechanism at a stated rate and rhythm (regular or irregular), and supplement this with an opinion about the most likely anatomic location of the abnormality, with or without proposed explanation for how it is sustained, e.g., "Supraventricular mechanism, rate 170, with regular rhythm, probably 'AV nodal reentrant tachycardia', less likely flutter with atrial rate 340. Atrial activity is not clear," or "Supraventricular mechanism, rate 170, probably junctional in origin and sustained by AV nodal reentry. Atrial activity is not identifiable." This approach has the advantage of leaving no doubt about the difference between what is seen and what it is thought to mean, but the considerable disadvantage of being cumbersome.

The importance of what name is chosen is less in cases in which the interpreter knows the clinical picture, and is the one who will determine management of the patient, than when the report is "on-line," when what one doctor says is going to be used by another to direct therapy. In the latter case, the arbitrary and changing nature of the names for ectopic tachycardias makes it especially important that there be good communication between the two.

Initiation of Ectopic Activity

Understanding of electrochemical events at the cell membrane level is still evolving, but in most instances the final common pathway to abnormality of function here, which can be identified clinically, is *ischemia*, and it can be assumed with confidence that all doctors understand *ischemia* to mean a local area of deficiency of blood, or, for practical purposes, of oxygen. The key word in that definition is *deficiency*, with its implication of inadequacy of supply as measured by need. Adequacy is related as much to demand as to supply, and to equate ischemia with impairment of flow, much less with the most common explanation for impairment of flow, is to assume more than is justified. The tracing shows abnormalities, not their etiology.

Factors that diminish the supply, considered collectively as "coronary insufficiency," are, usually, impairment of blood flow (the etymologic implication of the word), as with arterial stenosis due to atherosclerosis; loss of "vis à tergo," as with shock; or impairment of oxygen transfer, as with respiratory disease, but other possibilities exist. Increase in demand is brought about by increase in resistance to outflow from the affected area, exemplified, for atrial ectopy, by mitral valve disease, or, less obviously, by impairment of ventricular compliance as a result of overload, or by hypermetabolic states such as hyperpyrexia or hyperthyroidism. Anemia can be entered on both sides of the formula.

Other explanations include local change in electrophysiology, a *locus minoris resistentiae*, so that depolarization is provoked by events that normally would not have that effect. Some explanations for such a change are: trauma (including surgery), neoplastic implants (usually from breast or bronchus), inflammation (infection or infarction), drugs, and electrolyte imbalance. Information in the tracing makes it possible to specify the abnormality, but not what caused it.

Perpetuation of Ectopic Activity

The means by which ectopic activity is sustained is a subject for which explanations have been sought for nearly a hundred years. Several possibilities have been proposed, mostly variations on only two basic themes: repetitive activity inherent in a single focus, and some kind of a loop in which the wavefront set in motion by an impulse returns to initiate another. Clearly, both hypotheses have merit, and they may not be mutually exclusive. With so many options for intervention available, and with the logic of their application depending on the perception of how activity is sustained, this question still motivates the leading edge of investigation, and interest centers on reentry. Helpful as the surface EKG is, it is to electrophysiologic studies as light microscopy is to electron microscopy; not all information revealed by the more advanced method can be transferred directly to the less advanced one, but can often increase its value.

The earliest explanation for continuing ectopic activity, other than inherent automaticity associated with phase four depolarization, was known as *circus conduction*. It postulated a wave of excitation continuing about the junction of the venae cavae and the right atrium, and required features of repolarization and refractoriness that defined an "excitable gap," so that the advancing edge always found reactive tissue, characteristics not satisfied quantitatively in the normal heart. This "mother wave" gave rise somehow to "daughter" waves that spread centrifugally through the atria and died away at their peripheries. *Reentry* has been used almost as long to mean the same thing, and has all but replaced circus conduction in current parlance. The original concept of a long route around the base of the venae cavae was refuted in the 1940s by Prinzmetal and colleagues,[69] and the concept of "daughter waves" seems to have disappeared, but the basic idea, with details elaborated by intracardiac mapping, has survived. Not all reentry circuits require an anatomic obstacle as a nonreactive center, some may even be contained within the sinus or AV node or some other very small area.[70–73,577,704,705,711,918]

This logic is easy to follow in some instances, but much less so in others. It is not difficult, for instance, to picture an impulse spreading over the ventricles, and, reaching the periphery where it would be expected to end because there is nothing left to depolarize, finding instead an "alternative pathway," a Bundle of Kent, that allows it to continue into an atrium. If the atrial myocardium is responsive, the atria would be depolarized, the process would reenter the ventricles via normal channels, and so on endlessly. Details vary with the excitability of the myocardium, location and functional characteristics of the anomalous AV connection, rate, and other factors, but this is probably the means by which activity is sustained in the Wolff–Parkinson–White syndrome (p. 155). The EKG picture is characterized by a retrograde P following closely after a narrow QRS, sometimes continuous with it, and called *AV reentrant tachycardia* (p. 135).

The process now thought to explain classic flutter is known as *intraatrial reentry*, with the implication that the leading edge of a wave of excitation moves up one side of the atria and down the other so that atrial activity is indeed continuous. Almost by definition, this would make it impossible to call its projection on a lead to which it is nearly parallel either positive or negative, but it is not entirely parallel to any lead, and, given a firm definition of baseline, its projection in II, III, and aVF is negative. The fact that P waves may be discrete in other leads is not necessarily in conflict with the concept. Note that the events in this abnormality are confined to the atria; the AV junction functions normally, limiting the number of impulses that reach the ventricles to about 200/min, the same rate at which shortening of diastole begins to impinge significantly on ventricular filling, lessening the advantage to be gained by further increase in rate.

Some Special Characteristics and Terminology of the AV Junction Related to Abnormalities of Impulse Formation and Conduction

The junctional area is of importance in the genesis of tachycardias, and recordings from the His bundle and other parts of the intracardiac conduction system, begun in the late 1960s,[100–102] have demonstrated its complexity. The AV node itself is hard to pin down as an anatomic entity (p. 75), but its electrophysiologic properties have been studied extensively.[36–38,40] There may or may not exist another collection of cells with inherent automaticity just proximal to it, the *coronary sinus node*. There probably is more than one longitudinal pathway within the junction over which electrical wavefronts can travel at different rates and in different directions at the same time, but for most practical purposes it functions as a single channel, conducting from atria to ventricles.[33,411,891] *Longitudinal dissociation*[97,109–111,412,546] and *dual conduction*[111,112] within normal AV pathways may underlie *reentry.*[71,72,98,109–111,113–118,535]

The concept of *concealed conduction,*[103–105,425,426,461] incomplete penetration of atrial impulses into the AV node, has been offered as part of the explanation for the varying rate and rhythm of ventricular response to atrial fibrillation, and for prolongation of the PR in post-extrasystolic beats. *Exit block* is a complex concept implying failure of an impulse to be transmitted from its site of origin to surrounding tissues.[105,108,417,460]

The idea of *supernormal* conduction is controversial; its implication is that there are absolute and relative phases of reactivity just as there are of refractoriness. This hypothesis is invoked sometimes to explain unexpectedly short PR or narrow QRSs[119–122,425–427,898] (*see also* p. 147).

Default Mechanisms of Ventricular Origin

When impulses are not initiated by a faster, supraventricular pacemaker, or those that are are kept from reaching the ventricles, one within a ventricular wall will escape and drive them at a very slow rate, typically about 20–40/min, producing broad, bizarre QRSs with an approximately regular rhythm, an *idioventricular mechanism* (Fig. 8-5).

Patterns produced by *artificial pacemakers* (Fig. 8-5) vary with the position of the pacing electrode[370,371] and the features of the specific device as programmed, but two features can be recognized objectively—the pacemaker stimulus itself, and the complex it evokes. The stimulus appears as an instantaneous spike that may be positive or negative, great or small, depending on the position of the pacing electrode and the lead in which it is seen, and may or may not initiate a P or QRS, or fall within one. The characteristics of the paced complex depend on where the stimulus is introduced, those initiated in the right ventricle having the general form of left bundle branch block, and vice versa. Artificial pacemakers can pro-

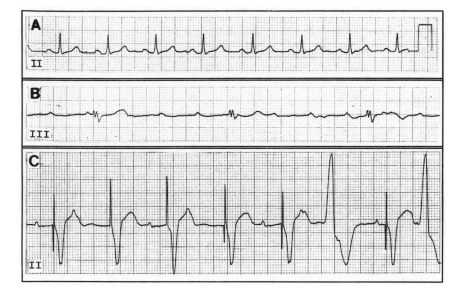

Fig. 8-5. Default mechanisms of ventricular origin. (**A**) is sinus for control. In (**B**) there is a sinus mechanism, rate 110, complicated by third degree AV block. The ventricles are driven from an intraventricular focus, rate about 30. In (**C**) there is a sinus mechanism, rate 100, third degree AV block, PVCs, and an artificial ventricular pacemaker firing and capturing appropriately, rate 75.

duce very complicated arrhythmias by interaction with intrinsic ones.[404] Distinction must be made between firing and capturing; a pacemaker may fire regularly without regards to intrinsic ventricular activity, or only when the cycle length exceeds a programmed figure, i.e., on demand, or unpredictably, and may capture appropriately, unpredictably, or not at all. Clinical application of findings requires that specific features of the pacemaker as programmed be known. Sometimes the pacemaker artifact itself may be mistaken for a QRS, but the absence of a T wave will point to proper identification.

Atrial standstill has been mentioned (p. 123), and there is such a thing, of course, as literal *cardiac standstill*, or cardiac arrest, manifest by a perfectly flat trace, no evidence of electrical activity.

Usurping Ventricular Mechanisms

The rate and rhythm of the ventricles can be determined easily, and the locus of the focus driving them is identified from the orientation, duration, amplitude, and contour of QRS, especially its duration and contour. If it is not wide, the impulse came from above the bifurcation of the bundle of His, and the beat is said to be of supraventricular origin; if wide and of bizarre configuration, it may have originated in the ventricular wall (spreading more slowly than normal, and following a course different from normal), or represent an intraventricular conduction defect (*see* p. 168 for the differential diagnosis of widening of QRS).

Premature Contractions

A premature ventricular contraction (PVC) produces a wide QRS with a configuration different from that of conducted beats in the same lead, appearing earlier than expected and not preceded by a conducted P wave[428,707,716] (Fig. 8-6). It originates within the ventricular wall, and, as with paced beats, the site is often implicit in its orientation and contour, those coming from the left ventricle having the form of right bundle branch block, and vice versa.[123] The ST-T pattern with PVCs is a combination of the original and change imposed on it by the altered route of depolarization. The pause between the premature beat and the conducted one that follows it is typically "compensatory"; i.e., the first post-extrasystolic beat occurs at the time it would have had there not been a PVC, but this is not always true, and a supraventricular premature beat also may be followed by a compensatory pause.

PVCs probably occur occasionally in everyone and, when asymptomatic and there is no myocardial disease, are unimportant, but, if they are frequent, arise from multiple foci, or, especially, if there is inflammatory myocardial disease (e.g., infarction), may require treatment.[124] There is a tradition that PVCs coinciding with the "vulnerable period" of ventricular repolarization (near the peak of T or on its return stroke) are likely to initiate ventricular automaticity, but there is reason to doubt this.[544] They may follow each con-

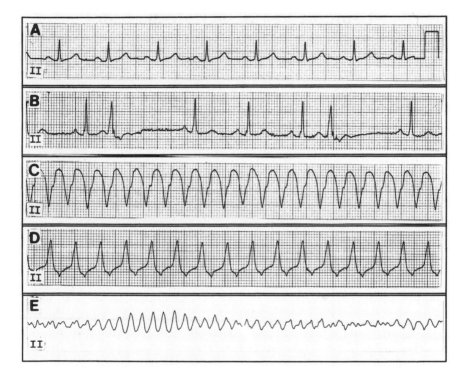

Fig. 8-6. Usurping mechanisms of ventricular origin. (**A**) is sinus for control, (**B**) shows premature ventricular contractions (PVCs), and in (**C**) there is ventricular tachycardia, rate 200. (**D**) shows ventricular tachycardia with retrograde P waves; and (**E**) ventricular fibrillation.

ducted beat, *ventricular bigeminy*, be sandwiched between two normal beats without breaking the regular rhythm, *interpolated PVCs* or true "extrasystoles," or occur after a P but before the impulse has had time to reach the ventricles, *end-diastolic PVCs*. In the latter case, if prematurity is not obvious, the presence of a normally timed P preceding the QRS makes recognition difficult. The PR interval of the first post-extrasystolic beat may be prolonged, and this may be related to such concepts as concealed retrograde conduction (p. 140). There may be various degrees of interaction between conducted impulses and those arising in the ventricular wall (*see fusion beats*, p. 169).

Ventricular Tachycardia

If a ventricular focus fires repetitively at a rapid rate, usually between 160–200, the mechanism is called *ventricular tachycardia* (Fig. 8-6), a name that implies two abnormalities, an ectopic focus and its rate. Differentiation from supraventricular tachycardia with bundle branch block, or other ventricular aberration, is important because of prognostic implications, but not always possible and the issue is often confused by use of the term "wide complex tachycardia." Control tracings, or control beats in the same tracing, help, and the clinical setting must always be taken into account in making an actionable decision. Several findings within the tracing are relevant. The presence of a usurping ventricular focus, for instance, does not mean that the sinus node ceases to function; demonstration of P waves at a rate slower than QRSs, with occasional conducted or fusion beats, is a major criterion for the diagnosis, but one that cannot always be demonstrated;[125,464] a situation much like that described as "interference dissociation" on p. 134. Retrograde depolarization of the atria from the ventricular focus occurs rarely.

It is traditional to describe ventricular rhythm as more likely to vary perceptibly with ventricular tachycardia than with supraventricular, and QRS configuration to be less consistent, but neither of these is always true. Recognition of ventricular ectopy is a particular problem in patients with pre-excitation, both because the Bundle of Kent offers an easy pathway for feedback to perpetuate what began as an otherwise innocent PAC or PVC, and because preexcitation itself both widens the QRS and alters its contour, simulating a ventricular origin.

Ventricular tachycardia is almost always evidence of important myocardial disease, but occurs, very rarely, in paroxysmal form, in the absence of other evidence of heart disease.[126] The means by which ventricular tachycardia is sustained is just as relevant as in supraventricular tachycardia, and the possibilities are similar, but it has not influenced the naming of the EKG picture nearly so much.

Occasionally one sees QRS complexes of ventricular origin at a rate greater than the usual escape rate of 30 or 40 but less than the 160 or more expected with ventricular tachycardia. There is no stan-

dard name for this, and such strange expressions as *slow ventricu-*
lar tachycardia, recurrent paroxysmal ventricular tachycardia,
accelerated idioventricular rhythm, and *ventricular tachysystole*
are found in the literature.[104,130,132] This problem is very similar to
the one that results in the term *accelerated junctional mechanism*
(p. 134). In each case, the locus is obvious, but the rate is not perceived
as either fast (tachy) or slow (brady). The temptation to Procrustean
thinking is avoided by simply following the rule to be as specific as
possible, naming the locus of the ectopic focus and giving its rate
and rhythm. The immediate clinical implication of these ventricular pacemakers of intermediate rate is less ominous than when the
rate is greater, but, like the faster ones, they define activity at the
lowest possible level; there is no backup.

Bidirectional Tachycardia

Bidirectional tachycardia is a rare finding characterized by broad,
bizarre QRS complexes of two configurations alternating with each
other.[432] One explanation for this is alternating block of anterior
and posterior divisions of the left bundle in the presence of right
bundle branch block[127] (p. 170).

Ventricular Flutter

Ventricular flutter has been mentioned from time to time as
something that would fit between ventricular tachycardia and ventricular fibrillation, but is a difficult and ill-defined concept with
little usefulness.

Ventricular Fibrillation

Ventricular fibrillation, often a terminal event, is seen rarely in
twelve-lead tracings, but commonly in monitoring units, and can
often be controlled. Ultimately, it produces a chaotic tracing with
no individually identifiable complexes (Fig. 8-6), but there is not a
point at which tachycardia ceases and fibrillation begins. These
catastrophic disorders may be simulated by muscle tremor, as paral-
ysis agitans, for instance, shivering from cold, chills, or fright, from

chest compression during attempts at resuscitation, or by technical artifacts such as loose attachment of electrodes, and have been known to be produced factitiously. Management of the patient always takes into account information in addition to that in the tracing. Like ventricular tachycardia, ventricular fibrillation has been documented as a paroxysmal event in otherwise normal young people,[128] and may be the basis for syncope in patients with long *QT syndromes* (*see* p. 234). One form of ventricular fibrillation, known as *torsades de pointes*, is a cyclic pattern in which the major direction of QRS shifts from positive to negative and back again, "twisting of the points." It is sometimes a paradoxical effect of antiarrhythmic drugs that prolong QT, including quinidine,[712,717,718,940] and other pharmacologic agents such as tricyclic antidepressants[713] and insecticides[714] (*see also* p. 184).

Miscellaneous

Bigeminy (literally, two twins) refers to pairing of beats, the repetitive occurrence of two beats relatively close together and separated from the next two by a longer interval. It may be explained by a premature beat (supraventricular or ventricular) after each beat of sinus origin, second degree AV block with 3:2 conduction, or other combinations. Escape–capture bigeminy is an unusual form in which a period of sinus inactivity results in escape of a lower pacemaker, followed by a sinus beat. To say only that the tracing shows bigeminy is not enough; the means by which the beats are paired must be given. It makes a difference whether pairing is due to premature discharge of an ectopic focus implying irritability, AV block implying depression of function, or compensatory mechanisms. Other recurring groupings of beats, as two PVCs following each sinus beat, for instance, are best described as such; "trigeminy" is an awkward term.

The idea of *parasystole* is that an ectopic pacemaker initiates beats at a rate slower than that of the sinus node, and is protected somehow from depolarization by sinus beats (*entrance block*[429]). Ventricular parasystole is the form most frequently recognized, but it occurs in the atria, too. It cannot be differentiated from ordinary premature beats unless suspected and the tracing is unusually long.[75,133–135,431,656,716] It may have no more clinical significance than any other premature beats.[418]

Supernormality of ventricular excitability may explain some ectopic beats in response to what otherwise would be an inadequate stimulus[667] (*see* p. 140).

NINE

Abnormalities
of Atrioventricular Conduction

The rate and rhythm of atria and ventricles can be noted objectively, but the origin of the impulses responsible for these features must be deduced from the characteristics of the curves they produce, and whether activity in the ventricles represents progression of an impulse from the atria, or vice versa, or they are unrelated, is always a judgment; the upper and lower hearts can interact in a variety of ways, and are capable of functioning independently. If there are both Ps and QRSs, a PR interval, defined simply as the distance between the beginning of P and the beginning of the next QRS, can be measured even when there is complete AV block. To record a figure for a PR interval is to express the opinion that the impulse responsible for atrial activity continued through the AV junction and depolarized the ventricles; all the tracing shows is Ps and QRSs.

Any lead in which both atrial and ventricular complexes can be seen, and is long enough to cover several heartbeats, will do for analysis of the mechanism. QRSs can almost always be recognized easily, but it's often hard to be sure about atrial activity; leads II and V1 are the ones usually best suited for this purpose, and an esophageal lead (p. 110), or even an intra-atrial one, can be used if necessary. In the very early days of electrocardiography, Lewis searched for P waves by pairing the arm leads in different positions on the chest while the lead selector switch was set at Lead I, an arrangement still mentioned sometimes as "Lewis leads." The mechanism, including AV block, is named in the context of the whole tracing, not individual groups of beats.

The normal relation between atrial and ventricular activity can be interrupted by either impairment of AV conduction, usurping atrial ectopy at a rate greater than the ability of the AV junction to conduct, or usurpation of pacemaker activity for the ventricles by an ectopic focus at a rate that renders them refractory to impulses transmitted normally from above. In each case, atria and ventricles are "disassociated," but, in practice, the phenomenon is identified by different names, if at all. In the first, AV block; the second, implicit in the diagnoses of the ectopic focus; and "AV dissociation" is used as if it were specific for the third.

AV Block

First degree AV block is present when PR is prolonged (Fig. 9-1); there is a QRS for each P, but it takes longer than normal for the impulse to get through the AV junction. The only problem here is to define the upper limit of normal for PR. PR is measured in the lead in which is longest *and* in which its beginning and end can be determined satisfactorily. It varies inversely with heart rate, and is also related to body size, ranging between 0.16 s, in small adults with rates above 130, to 0.21 s in large ones with rates below 70,[934] figures that are enlightening but hard to apply clinically. With the beginning of QRS, the B point, as a given, the limiting factor is assignment of a point for the origin of P, and this is arbitrary (p. 27). A PR of 0.20 s, like a blood pressure of 120, is about what would be expected, not the upper limit of normal with the implication that any greater figure, even 0.21 s, as read by a computer program, is abnormal. As heart rate increases, so does the problem of defining prolongation of PR; first degree AV block is rarely diagnosed at rates above 100, and not at all when there is atrial tachycardia. AV conduction is often normal with sinus activity at rates that would produce second degree AV block if the pacemaker were in an atrium (p. 130), and this may be evidence of its enhancement by the increased production of catecholamines often associated with sinus tachycardia (p. 154). The duration of PR is a statistic whose significance to the patient can be assessed only in clinical context. Borderline values are common in healthy people, and, as an incidental finding, are of little if any importance (p. 236).[840,841] The longer the PR, the more likely it is to be evidence of significant abnormality,

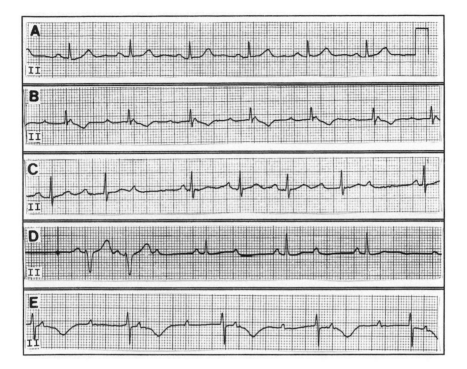

Fig. 9-1. Atriventricular block. (**A**) shows a sinus mechanism with normal AV conduction. In (**B**) PR is about 0.32 s, first degree AV block; in (**C**) PR lengthens progressively until a QRS is dropped, and the cycle starts again, second degree AV block, Type I, or Wenckebach; and in (**D**) PR is constant and normal in the first two beats, but no QRS follows the third, Type II, or Mobitz, second degree AV block. In this example, there is an IV conduction defect in the first two beats, and this resolves when the interval between QRSs is longer. In (**E**) AV block is complete and there is a junctional pacemaker for the ventricles, rate 45.

but even marked prolongation may be benign, and does not necessarily predict more advanced degrees of block.[733,734]

First degree AV block is not a disease, but may be perceived as one, especially if it is called *heart block*, and this is one of the insidious risks a patient accepts when he or she has an electrocardiogram made. The effect of such an interpretation on insurance programs, job security, and happiness is hard to predict. If first degree AV block is present and significant, it is an important finding and must be named, but to call it on estimates of 0.01 s, or, even worse, to accept a computer readout as meaningful without question, is to fail to recognize the limits of the method.

Second degree AV block is present when all QRSs are initiated by atrial activity but not all atrial activity is followed by QRSs. Atrial activity is usually in the form of Ps, so in most cases this translates to fewer QRSs than Ps, all QRSs preceded by Ps but not all Ps followed by QRSs. When there is atrial fibrillation, there is always second degree AV block (i.e., all ventricular activity is initiated by atrial activity, but not all atrial impulses are followed by ventricular response), and it is not listed as a separate entity.

Given a sinus mechanism, there are two types of second degree AV block, Types I and II (Fig. 9-1). In Type I, the PR interval increases progressively until a P is blocked completely and there is a P wave without a following QRS. The next PR is short, and the cycle repeats, the Wenckebach phenomenon. The number of beats in a cycle may be fixed or variable. In Type II, PR does not vary; QRSs are dropped unpredictably. When every other QRS is dropped, distinction between Types I and II is arbitrary. Both types were described by both Wenckebach and Mobitz, but Type I is commonly known by Wenckebach's name and Type II by Mobitz's. It is interesting that Wenckebach's description was based on recordings of jugular and apical pulses before electrocardiography was available.[860]

To equate second degree AV block with impairment of AV conduction fails to separate description from interpretation. The definition proposed above is intended to be as precise as possible; it carefully refers to impulses from the atria, not only P waves but also f waves, and is limited to information from the tracing; explanation for it is left for clinical judgment. When the atrial rate is below about 180, second degree AV block means impairment of AV conduction; above that rate, it demonstrates the normal filtering effect of the node. The normal AV junction cannot conduct more than about 180–200 beats/min, the same rate at which short-

ening of diastole begins to impinge on the rapid phase of ventricular filling, and this has the effect of protecting the ventricles from
an inefficiently rapid rate. One advantage of limiting the definition
of second degree AV block to an objective statement of events documented in the tracing, not including an explanation for them, is
apparent when atrial flutter is considered (p. 129).

Third degree, or complete, AV block implies that none of the
impulses from above reaches the ventricles, which must be driven
by a focus below the block (Fig. 9-1). The electrocardiogram shows
QRSs at a rate slower than atrial, with a regular rhythm, and no
predictable relation between the two. When the pacemaker below
the block is junctional, QRS complexes are narrow (unless there is
also an IV conduction defect), and typically at a rate of about 40 to
50; when it is in a ventricle (*idioventricular*), broad, slurred, of
bizarre configuration, and at a rate of about 20 to 30. QRS rhythm
is regular in both cases. Junctional pacemakers are likely to be stable;
idioventricular ones, unstable.

Discussion

The electrocardiographic diagnosis of AV block is not difficult
if the tracing is long enough for adequate study and atrial complexes can be identified with confidence. Organization of the information in the form of a diagram is helpful in separating atrial from
ventricular activity (Fig. 8-1, p. 121).[698] One advantage of an EKG
format of three simultaneous leads is that atrial activity may be
visible from one view while not from another, and an additional
unbroken "rhythm strip," usually Lead II, avoids pattern change
with lead changes.

AV block may result from a combination of lesions in the IV
conduction system or from a single lesion in the His Bundle or
above.[101] It is commonly a result of inflammatory disease (infection
or infarction), drugs (quinidine and other antiarrhythmics, or, especially, digitalis), or anatomic lesions of whatever cause,[138,148] but
may be seen as an incidental finding in otherwise healthy subjects
(p. 236), and with sleep apnea (p. 237). It may be congenital, usually in association with other lesions such as an endocardial cush-

ion defect or corrected transposition of the great vessels, but this is uncommon.[146,407,408] The fixed, chronic, complete AV block of elderly patients with or without dizzy spells, syncope, or seizures, Stokes–Adams attacks, is usually idiopathic. Complete block as a result of drugs is rare. The electrocardiogram shows only the block, not its etiology.

AV Dissociation

In the discussion above, all the examples of AV block reflect impaired function of the junctional apparatus, but there is another way supraventricular impulses can be kept from entering the ventricles. Physiologic refractoriness of the conducting tissues or myocardium has the same effect, and this occurs when an ectopic focus drives the ventricles at a rate greater than sinus. In both cases, atria and ventricles function independently, i.e., are disassociated, but in common practice this is called AV block when attributed to impairment of a normal function, AV conduction, and "AV dissociation" when resulting from excess of a different one, automaticity, as if the generic term excluded the specific. It is not named at all when it is part of the picture of atrial flutter, atrial fibrillation, or ventricular tachycardia (*see also accelerated junctional mechanisms*, p. 134).

Short PR

There are several ways PR may be shortened, but no useful figure for the lower limit of normal can be given; 0.12 s is not unusual in healthy subjects, and values below that are hard to estimate. Conduction velocity may be enhanced by catecholamines,[36,732] but not much else. Abnormal shortening is more likely because of bypass of the AV node via tracts that communicate directly with the His Bundle,[181,650,708,743,744] or enter the ventricular myocardium at some peripheral site, and there may be such a thing as supernormal AV conduction (p. 140). The time between P and QRS may be short when there is isorhythmic dissociation (p. 134), but in this case the QRS does not represent progression of the impulse that produced the P; there is no true PR interval (p. 149).

Ventricular Pre-Excitation

If the impulse from the atria bypasses the AV node, entering the ventricular myocardium via one of several other possible pathways,[439] QRS will begin early, and the contour of the initial part may or may not be changed. The classic example of this is the electrocardiographic part of a syndrome described in 1930 by Wolff, Parkinson, and White[179] in "healthy young adults and children with apparently normal hearts" who had histories of "tachycardia or auricular fibrillation." Other explanations have been proposed, but the overwhelming evidence is that it is a result of passage of atrial impulses to ventricles through anomalous conduction tissue, a Bundle of Kent, at some peripheral site.[180–195] When the ventricles are "pre-excited" by this means, the early wavefront merges with that from normal pathways to produce a fusion beat (p. 169). This is manifest by an early slur in QRS, called a *delta wave* because of its fancied resemblance to the upstroke of the Greek letter.[696] QRS is widened, and PR is shortened; the time from beginning of P to end of QRS is not changed. The QRS pattern may be divided into two groups on the basis of QRS orientation: in Type A, it is directed anteriorly and either superiorly or inferiorly, and may simulate right bundle branch block (Fig. 9-2); in Type B, to the left, posterior, and either superior or inferior, simulating left bundle branch block (Fig. 9-3). There is little if any clinical value in differentiating between these, especially now that the abnormal pathway can be located precisely, but there is some evidence that atrial fibrillation may be more frequent in patients with the Type A pattern.[932] The QRS-T angle is almost always wide with pre-excitation; i.e., T is negative in leads with positive QRS, but the ST-T pattern varies with the location of the anomalous tissue and its conductive characteristics.

Ventricular pre-excitation occurs in about 0.15 percent of the population,[19,185] and in all age groups, probably most frequently in young adults. It is an incidental finding in many instances, but is commonly associated with paroxysmal supraventricular tachycardia,[180,186] presumably because of the opportunity for circulation of the excitatory process provided by the presence of a conducting pathway between atria and ventricles in addition to the normal one. The diagnostically critical early QRS slur, the delta wave, often

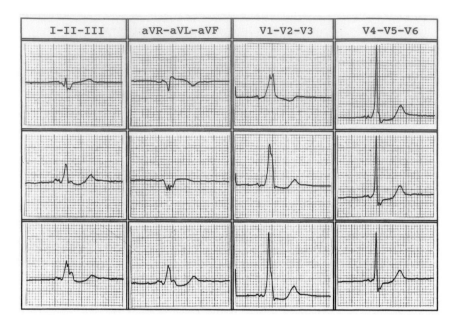

Fig. 9-2. Ventricular pre-excitation, Type A.

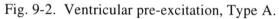
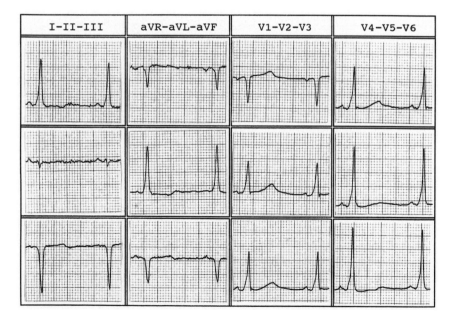

Fig. 9-3. Ventricular pre-excitation, Type B.

disappears during paroxysms of tachycardia. When QRS distortion persists during tachycardia, it may be nearly impossible to differentiate from bundle branch block, with which it may coexist,[187] or ventricular tachycardia,[188] the predominantly initial location of the slur being the only key. The problem of diagnosis is even greater if there is atrial fibrillation. The presence of the accessory pathway may not only produce a QRS pattern that simulates ventricular ectopy, but also may precipitate it. Pre-excitation can either simulate or obscure evidence of myocardial infarction,[189-192] and may be persistent or remarkably labile, present in some tracings and not in others, or even in alternate beats in the same tracing. In some cases it may be made to appear or disappear in response to changes in vagus tone, exercise, position, or even deep breathing.[180] The EKG response to exercise in patients with Wolff–Parkinson–White syndrome is almost always "positive."[332,735]

Patients with ventricular pre-excitation have benefited more than any other group from the new discipline of clinical electrophysiology. Recordings from selected positions within atria and ventricles have made it possible to study the effect of drugs on response to controlled electrical stimuli, and to locate accessory pathways precisely enough to permit their ablation by surgery,[193,194,406] or, most recently, electrocoagulation via cardiac catheter techniques.[950]

The Lown–Ganong–Levine Syndrome, short PR with normal QRS and a history of paroxysmal rapid heart action, especially common in middle aged women, is not diagnosed from the tracing alone. It implies bypass of the AV node by way of anomalous pathways other than a Bundle of Kent.[181,648-650,743,819]

TEN

Abnormalities
of Intraventricular Conduction

Impairment of intraventricular conduction produces changes in orientation, duration, amplitude, and/or contour of QRS. Specific patterns depend on the location and extent of the lesion, and can be predicted with confidence from the anatomic and physiologic properties of the system summarized in Chapter Four (p. 75).

Right Bundle Branch Block

Interruption of conduction in the right bundle branch does not interfere with depolarization of the left side of the IV septum and the left ventricle, but delays activation of the right ventricle, requiring it to follow a path different from normal, at a rate slower than normal, writing the last part of QRS after the left ventricle, or most of it, has been depolarized. This is expressed as a broad, slurred terminal wave in QRS directed to the right and anteriorly, an S in lead I and an R in V1. The QRS duration is at least 0.12 s (Fig. 10-1).

The right ventricle is more anterior than right, and the abnormal terminal R in V1 is more stable evidence of right bundle branch block than the S in Lead I.[816,832] This pattern merges with that of right ventricular enlargement on the one hand, and with normal on the other. An rSr in V1 may be found in any of these, and to imply abnormality by calling it "incomplete right bundle branch block" is of little value.[555]

Orientation of the frontal QRS as a whole, its axis, is not a criterion for the diagnosis of right bundle branch block,[171,172] but when right bundle branch block is present it is especially important to remember that the axis is a function of area, not amplitude alone, and of the whole QRS, not its initial or terminal parts selectively.

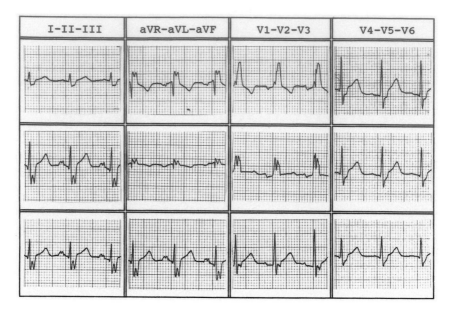

Fig. 10-1. Right bundle branch block.

Very often in Lead I the initial R is taller than the terminal S is deep, but S is so much broader than R that the net area is negative; the mean frontal QRS is directed to the right, but systems that consider only the amplitude will call it left.

In the absence of other disease, the T wave of right bundle branch block is of normal contour and directed opposite the blocked part of QRS, negative in right precordial leads and positive in left, substantially the same as when QRS is normal. When there is associated myocardial disease, e.g., patchy fibrosis, primary ST-T abnormalities may be superimposed.

Left Bundle Branch Block

Unlike the right bundle branch, a slender strand through most of its course, like a wire, the left one is a literal bundle, like a cable, that begins to become frayed shortly after its origin at the bifurcation at the Bundle of His, an anatomic characteristic that explains differences in the EKG evidence of left and right bundle branch block. Block of the right branch produces a pattern that varies in detail but always includes a broad, slurred, terminal component directed anteriorly and, usually, to the right, but that owing to block in the left system depends on its specific location. If it is proximal enough, the route of excitation of the interventricular septum, as well as that, of the free wall of the left ventricle, is changed. The typical result, in a lead in which QRS is positive, is a complex at least 0.12 s in duration with a brisk upstroke, a notched top, and rapid return to the baseline (Fig. 9-2). This is the prototype of "complete," or proximal, left bundle branch block; axis is not a criterion,[660,831,834] but the complex is usually directed to the left, caudad and dorsad. If the block is slightly more distal, initial QRS forces may not be changed, and this is relevant when the question of a myocardial infarct arises in a patient whose tracing shows left bundle branch block (pp. 170, 183).

The T wave in uncomplicated left bundle branch block is of normal contour but directed opposite to QRS, but coexisting myocardial disease may change its direction, amplitude, or contour.

Block of Subdivisions of the Left Bundle

One of the most important developments in electrocardiography in the 1960s was recognition that the left bundle branch can be considered as dividing, shortly after its origin, into at least two, and probably three, groups of fibers, or fascicles—anterior, posterior, and anteroseptal.[534,540,543] The early work of Grant,[159] Pryor and Blount,[160] and Watt et al.[161] should be noted, James's studies were of fundamental importance,[507] and the contributions of Rosenbaum were especially influential.[151,164,451] The existence of these fascicles as discrete entities is still controversial, but in the present state of knowledge they are reasonable and useful explanations for findings that are enigmatic otherwise. The nomenclature of conduction delay in these subdivisions is inconsistent, but not very important; *hemiblock*, left anterior and left posterior, is used widely, but *fas-*

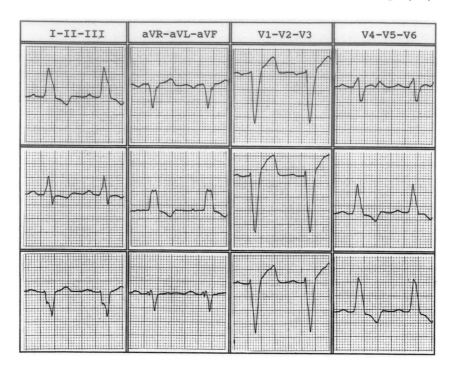

| I–II–III | aVR–aVL–aVF | V1–V2–V3 | V4–V5–V6 |

Fig. 10-2. Left bundle branch block.

cicular block is more logical because it leaves room for more than two components; both terms are in common use. Gradation between proximal, or complete, left bundle branch block, and block of its subdivisions, is a continuum,[508] and, by whatever name, the implication is that there is a local lesion in the conduction system that interferes with its function.

Left Anterior Fascicular Block

In subjects without heart disease, the frontal QRS axis lies between about −30 and +105°. Positions outside this range, abnormal by definition, may be the result of any of several processes including change in the electrical properties of the system, technical error, thoracic deformity, ectopic origin of QRS, and the effects of drugs and electrolytes (p. 226). There is a group of patients, however, whose QRS is directed to between −45 and −90° and in whom none of these explanations is applicable. It is hypothesized that, in these subjects, activation of the anterosuperior part of the ventricular myocardium, directed leftward and upward, is delayed, occurring after that in the opposite wall of the ventricles, rightward and inferiorly, has been completed. The terminal part of QRS reflects this imbalance by being oriented more leftward and superiorly than normal. An anatomic basis for such a lesion has been established by the demonstration of subdivisions of the left bundle branch,[164,507] but study of such small structures is exceedingly difficult, and there are differences of opinion over the extent to which they are functionally distinct. That they are, that there is such a thing as fascicular block, is supported by several observations. Scarification of the ventricular myocardium of primates in areas predicated to include anterior superior ramifications of the left bundle branch has been shown to produce the expected electrocardiographic changes,[161] and the picture has been noted during left anterior descending coronary artery opacification[167] and during graded exercise testing.[531] Also, it occurs sometimes as a transient finding in association with chest pain typical of angina, and following coronary artery surgery.

What all this amounts to is that direction of the frontal QRS, to between −45 and −90°, with normal initial contour, and in the absence of some other explanation for it, can be interpreted as evidence of impairment of conduction in the anterior superior ramification of the left bundle branch, i.e., left anterior fascicular block. QRS duration may be prolonged but, this is not necessary for the diagnosis (Fig. 10-3).

The presence of left anterior fascicular block, as with any IV conduction defect, identifies a lesion in the ventricular wall but does not suggest what caused it or whether it will persist or be transient. Local impairment of oxygen supply by coronary atherosclerosis is high on the list of probable explanations, of course, but other possibilities include endocardial cushion defect, trauma, infection, infiltrative disease, edema, drug effect, and metabolic change;[661,663] proof of the cause is rarely forthcoming, and distinction from normal is often arbitrary. It is common in older people and may mean that there is patchy fibrosis in the myocardium,[451] but, as an incidental find-

I–II–III	aVR–aVL–aVF	V1–V2–V3	V4–V5–V6

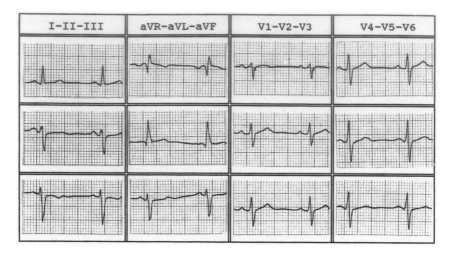

Fig. 10-3. Left anterior fascicular block.

ing, need not be of clinical importance. It may be produced by a myocardial infarct, but it may also simulate[511,538,691] or obscure one.[164]

The question of how to recognize *left anterior fascicular block in the presence of an inferior infarct, and vice versa*, is an interesting one. They may coexist, of course, but to diagnose both from a single tracing involves conflict. "Left axis deviation" is necessary for the diagnosis of left anterior fascicular block, but can be explained also by loss of rightward and downward forces as with an inferior infarct; one of the criteria for left anterior fascicular block is normality of the initial part of QRS, but the diagnosis of infarction rests upon its abnormality. If normality of the initial forces is not included as necessary for the diagnosis of left anterior fascicular block, the only requirement is the direction of the terminal ones, "left axis deviation," and, if this is explained by an inferior infarct, it cannot be used again to mean something else at the same time.[621,715,752,753] A similar, but less prominent, problem is encountered in making the diagnosis of *left ventricular hypertrophy and left anterior fascicular block* from the same tracing; the abnormal axis may be evidence of either an increase in muscle mass or of left anterior hemiblock due to patchy fibrosis that often accompanies hypertrophy. Pulmonary emphysema may simulate left anterior fascicular block by invalidating Einthoven's premise of equal conductivity (p. 232), and potassium toxicity may produce a very similar picture (p. 231).

Left Posterior Fascicular Block

Left posterior fascicular block is diagnosed rarely. It probably occurs less frequently than the anterior lesion because of the more generous blood supply in the postero-inferior region of the septum from both left and right coronary arteries, and because its more diffuse nature makes block unlikely.[164,169] Criteria for its diagnosis are: a mean frontal QRS more clockwise than +105°, and, usually, a small initial R in Lead I and Q in II and III (Fig. 10-4). As with anterior hemiblock, it may result from anything that impairs conduction, but distinction from normal on the one hand and from right ventricular enlargement on the other is usually arbitrary. Its presence with acute myocardial infarction has been correlated with a poor prognosis.[762]

Anterior Septal Fascicular Block

There is reason to suspect that an anterior septal subdivision of the left bundle branch exists as a functional entity, and that block of it produces a prominent R wave in V1.[534,540,541,543,580,623] If there is such a fascicle, the *hemiblock* and *trifascicular* terminology is not accurate.

Other Explanations for Abnormally Tall R in V1

Other explanations for abnormally tall R in V1 include right ventricular hypertrophy, right bundle branch block, and dorsal myocardial infarction. Left ventricular hypoplasia may produce a similar picture, and so may asymmetric septal hypertrophy.[452] Technical error must be considered: transposition of V1 and a lead from farther to the left, or the lead labeled V1 is plugged into the slot for V4, say, so that what the machine records as V1 is really V4.

Combinations of Intraventricular Blocks

During the same time that subdivision of the left bundle branch into two fascicles was giving rise to the concept of a trifascicular conduction system, artificial ventricular pacing was becoming pos-

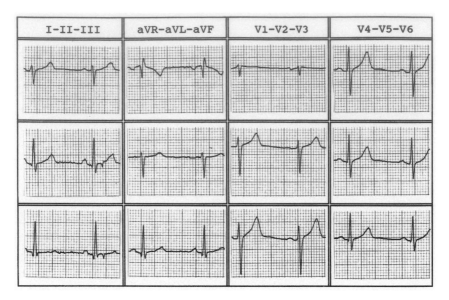

Fig. 10-4. Left posterior fascicular block.

sible, and the idea developed, logically, that block of half of the left bundle branch in a patient with right bundle branch block might presage complete AV block and, thus, be an indication for prophylactic pacing. The consequences to the patient of such reasoning are so important that the hypothesis must be examined carefully. It presents two problems: First, is it possible to make the diagnosis of block at two sites from a single set of data when each lesion is expressed as abnormality of the same part of the QRS selectively; and second, even if this can be done, does the prognosis of asymptomatic patients with this combination justify the risk of such major intervention?

There is no doubt that block of the right bundle branch occurs and can be identified, it is easy to accept the hypothesis that block of only part of the left bundle produces a characteristic EKG picture as well, and there is no reason to doubt that both may be present in the same heart, but to identify both in a single tracing is another matter. One of the fascicles of "bifascicular block" is always the right bundle branch, and the other is almost always the anterior subdivision of the left; the posterior one is invoked rarely. The premise that both blocks can be recognized in a single tracing is based on the assumption that, when the uncontroversial and easily recognized pattern of right bundle branch block (in which axis is not a factor) is present, and there is also "left axis deviation," there must also be left anterior hemiblock.[150,151] The difficulty here is that each lesion is manifest in the terminal portion of QRS selectively. In right bundle branch block there is, typically, a terminal S in Lead I; i.e., the terminal forces are directed to the right, but marked leftward direction of these same forces is a *sine qua non* for the diagnosis of left anterior fascicular block.

The problem stems from conflict in application of two of the most basic premises of electrocardiography: The trace represents the position of a single point in space, and simultaneous radial depolarization of the ventricles is normal. The presence of right bundle branch block is an announcement that the ventricles are not being depolarized simultaneously, that one of the assumptions on which the recognition of left anterior fascicular block is based has been invalidated. Less fundamental, but equally important, is the meaning of "axis deviation" (p. 226); i.e., how axis is determined, the limits of the method, and the range of normal. Both of the lesions in question affect terminal forces only; should the initial part of the complex be considered? Also, the idea that left axis deviation in the presence of right bundle branch block means that there is left anterior fascicular block is not defensible; however one chooses to define "left axis deviation," several explanations for it are possible (p. 226).

Bifascicular block is a convincing term, and an altogether reasonable hypothesis, but recognition of it in a single tracing depends on estimation of very, very small values, reasoning that is open to question, and is probably beyond the limits of the method. If the diagnosis of left anterior fascicular block has been established, the addition of right bundle branch block in later tracings can be recognized easily, and the diagnosis of both is probably justifiable, if next to impossible to prove, but this requires more than one tracing and is of questionable prognostic value. Several studies have failed to show that patients with right bundle branch block and left axis deviation (by various criteria) are significantly more likely to develop third degree AV block than other members of the population.[518,522,526,548,647,761]

If the question of temporary prophylactic pacing arises in a patient already in a monitoring facility, it is not nearly so difficult to resolve; facilities for pacing are immediately at hand, and the procedure involves only transient discomfort and little added expense, not commitment to permanent pacing. The elderly patient with right bundle branch block and "left axis deviation" who is to undergo surgery, but has no clinical heart disease, presents another special case. Here temporary pacing may be justified on the basis of doing no harm and perhaps being life saving, but prospective studies have indicated that even in this setting the risk of the pacemaker is greater than its benefit.[548]

AV block may result from a combination of lesions distal to the bifurcation of the Bundle of His,[136] but the concept of "bilateral bundle branch block" is ill defined and seems to imply simply complete AV block. The nature of the tracing, that it reflects the motion of a single point, is in conflict with its showing the patterns of both left and right bundle branch block at the same time.[144,177,178] The typical pattern of IV block may result from local lesions above the bifurcation,[546] but it still is not possible to identify these without the aid of special intracardiac recording techniques.[101]

Other Explanations for Widening of QRS

Abnormality of intraventricular conduction is usually fixed, but may be *intermittent*,[212,213] found in some tracings and not in others, or even in some beats and not others in the same tracing, and there are several means, other than block of a bundle branch, complete or partial, by which prolongation of QRS may be brought about. When attributed to lesions distal to the main branches, it has been called *arborization block*[16] and *parietal block*,[195] but neither of these is accepted now as meaningful. *Peri-infarction block* has never been very clearly defined. It is not an entity in itself, but has been proposed as an explanation for QRS prolongation, as well as change in terminal forces, sometimes seen in tracings that show an infarct. Apparently the earliest rationale for this is still the most likely one, delay of impulse transmission by detour around the lesion, and/or by impairment of conduction through surviving fibers within it. *Left anterior fascicular block*, now accepted as an entity itself, is probably what Grant was describing when he used the term[14,164,196–198,816,833,895] (*see also* p. 184).

Sometimes, in tracings in which most QRS complexes are narrow, broad ones occur, either singly or in groups, and the question of ventricular ectopy arises. These beats may reflect transient modification of the route of depolarization as a result of refractoriness of conduction tissue, *ventricular aberration*.[199,201,459,540,577] Their configuration is usually that of right bundle branch block. Aberration is common when a supraventricular beat follows closely upon another, as with PACs, atrial tachycardia, flutter, and fibrillation. The most important reason to recognize it is the difference in prognosis between atrial and ventricular ectopy. *Fusion beats* reflect merger of two wavefronts, a normally conducted one and one from a PVC, for instance, producing a QRS that is not characteristic of either alone but includes elements of both.[444] This is probably the explanation for the deformity typical of *ventricular pre-excitation* (p. 155). *Drugs*, especially quinidine and other antiarrhythmics, and tricyclic antidepressants (p. 230), can prolong the QRS without change in configuration, and *hyperkalemia* (p. 231) has the same general effect. *Paper speed of 50 mm/s* can make the QRS seem wide when it is not, and a P wave that overlaps QRS, especially common in atrial flutter (p. 130) and in high and low junctional mechanisms, may be read mistakenly as part of QRS.

Summary and Comment

Block of either the right or the left branch of the bundle of His is the most common form of intraventricular conduction delay. It is recognized by prolongation of the QRS to 0.12 s or more with the terminal forces directed toward the side of the block. Whether block of a subdivision of the left bundle branch can be recognized is controversial, but there is experimental and clinical evidence to support the idea, and it is a useful hypothesis. Intraventricular block has no clinical manifestations itself; its importance is that it is evidence of a lesion not otherwise identifiable. It may be caused by coronary atherosclerosis, trauma,[205] infection, or any other cause of myocardial disease, and may be congenital.[206]

Bundle Branch Block
and Myocardial Infarction

Recognition of a myocardial infarct in the presence of right bundle branch block presents no problem; the infarct shows in the proximal part of QRS which is not affected. Block of the left bundle branch, if proximal enough to distort the initial part of QRS, may mask evidence of an infarct, but if the criteria for both are fulfilled, both may be recognized in the same tracing.[192,207,208,478] In either case, an infarct and bundle branch block are separate entities in no conflict; either may be present without the other. The diagnosis of bundle branch block is an objective interpretation of findings in the tracing without speculation regarding their cause or effect, but to say that there is an infarct is not only to interpret them but also to explain them.

Bundle Branch Block
and Ventricular Hypertrophy

Bundle branch block and ventricular hypertrophy may coexist, but depolarization of the ventricles out of phase invalidates the base for the criteria for hypertrophy; the two cannot be diagnosed from a single tracing with confidence.[209–211,442] The diagnosis of hypertrophy of the opposite ventricle in the presence of bundle branch block is especially tenuous. Diagnosis of an intraventricular conduction defect identifies a local lesion in the wall of the ventricle, but does not suggest an explanation for it; Enlargement, dilatation, hypertrophy, and overload all imply response to a hemodynamic burden.

An IV conduction defect may be *rate dependent*, either fast or slow,[214–216,481,490,658] and may be an apparently benign finding.[217,401] *Alternation* of the patterns of right and left bundle branch block, either beat to beat or tracing to tracing, seems to identify advanced but unstable delay in conduction of both systems. In patients with syncope, it suggests that complete AV block is imminent,[933] but examples of its persistence for years without progression have been known.[659] Bundle branch block has been reported as hereditary,[541] and has been found in healthy athletes.[19,824] It does not produce serious hemodynamic consequences,[450] but may cause wide splitting of the first heart sound and, in the case of left bundle branch, paradoxical splitting of the second one.

ELEVEN

Myocardial Infarction

Perhaps the most conspicuous of all the uses of electrocardiography, well known to patients as well as doctors, is for evaluation of chest pain, and indeed it can be very helpful, especially when myocardial infarction is suspected. It can suggest the diagnosis, support it, or fail to support it, but can never, by itself, either establish it or rule it out. The diagnosis of an infarct says not only that there is an area of dead tissue deep in the myocardium, but also what caused it to die; the tracing can show the lesion, its location, and, with certain assumptions, how long it has been there, but not what caused it. Other explanations for each of the findings typical of an infarct, and for all of them together, are possible, and there may be no identifiable EKG evidence of even an acute one.

Criteria for Recognition of an Infarct

Changes that would be expected to occur in an EKG as a result of an infarct are just what would be predicted on the basis of well-known features of anatomy and physiology.

1. The blood supply to the myocardium enters superficially and ramifies deep;
2. Depolarization of the ventricular wall proceeds outward from the endocardium; and
3. Tissue at the distal end of the system suffers first when blood flow is diminished.
4. If deficiency of blood supply is severe enough for long enough, the tissue dies, is infarcted; and
5. Dead tissue is electrically inactive.
6. Absence of electrical activity in one part of the myocardium, although normal in the rest, changes the net result of the process.

It follows that an infarct, a wedge-shaped lesion with its base distal to the point of arterial compromise, modifies forces generated early in the process of depolarization, producing change in the first part of QRS.

There are exceptions to each these points and much overlap between normal and abnormal at each step, but the logic they describe is valid. Not all infarcts can be recognized electrocardiographically, but when one can, the *sine qua non* is abnormality of the initial part of QRS. Because of the polarity and positioning of the leads with relation to the heart, this is usually in the form of an abnormal Q,[229,909,910] an *abnormal* Q, not just a Q, and the characteristics of normal must be understood before abnormal can be identified.

Abnormality of the Initial Part of QRS

The initial component of a typical, normal QRS (pp. 41, 91) is directed to the right, cephalad, and anterior, producing a Q in leads I, aVL, and V6 whose most important features are its duration and contour; a *normal* Q is narrow, not more than about 0.03 s in duration, and "clean," sharp angles and straight lines. Orientation is indicated by the name "Q" *and* the lead in which it is seen, and amplitude is not very important.

There are *two ways a Q wave can be abnormal*: intrinsically, and by location. First, its *intrinsic* features, duration and contour. It is easy to define 0.03 s as the upper limit of normal for duration, but to call it this close, to a quarter of a millimeter, is clearly beyond the limit of the method. Contour is being assessed at the same time, though, and the combination of wide and "dirty" (notched, jagged) is what determines abnormality, a judgment that cannot be quantified completely.

Second, *location*: No matter how clean and narrow it may be, a Q where a Q does not belong is abnormal. Criteria for where one belongs can be given easily for precordial leads, but not for frontal ones. Beginning with V1 and progressing toward V6, the first time a Q appears it will initiate a predominantly positive QRS, and it will not grow smaller (relative to the following R) in leads made farther to the left. Criteria for a normal R in precordial leads are similar;

moving from V1 toward V6, the first time an R appears it will initiate the QRS, and it will not grow smaller (relative to the following S) in leads made farther to the left. These features cannot be quantified precisely, but to think of the amplitude of the Q, or initial R, as a proportion of the following wave is helpful; RV6 is often smaller than RV5, for instance, and electrodes are seldom placed in exactly the same spots in serial tracings (Fig. 11-1).

Examples

A clean, sharp QS is found commonly in V1 and V2 in normals, and may be seen even farther to the left, but a QS in V2 is abnormal if there is an rS in V1. A QS in V1–2 followed by an Rs in V3 is normal, but a QS in V1–2 followed by a qrS in V3 is likely to be evidence of an infarct. These patterns have given rise to the expression "poor progression of the R wave,"[746,747] but it is the initial part of the QRS that must be considered, not just the R wave, and it is possible to describe the findings much more objectively than "poor."

An early slur or notch on the downstroke of a QS in V1 may be the only evidence of an anterior infarct, or an initial R in V1 of a dorsal one, but neither of these is enough to make much of as an isolated, incidental finding.

Similar rules for defining abnormality of the initial part of QRS in leads II, III, and aVF, especially III, for recognition of an inferior infarct (Fig. 11-2) are not possible. The same standards apply as in the anterior leads, but most forces produced in ventricular depolarization in most people are nearly perpendicular to the line of Lead III. Tiny changes in direction, not detectable in leads to which the forces are nearly parallel, can make the difference between positive and negative in lead III, and QRS is likely to be small and transitional there as well. More interpretation is necessary in recognizing inferior lesions than anterior ones. Abnormality of the initial part of QRS is still critical, but it is not the only factor; the ST-T pattern, change from control, and the clinical setting are all to be considered. These factors, not any feature intrinsic in computers, explain why computer programs are so good at recognizing anterior infarcts and so unreliable with inferior ones.

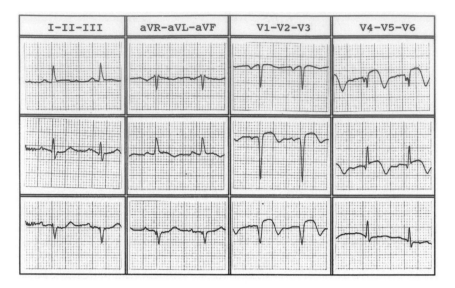

Fig. 11-1. Acute anterior myocardial infarct.

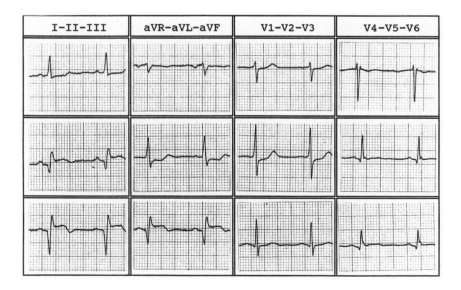

Fig. 11-2. Acute inferior myocardial infarct.

Origin of the Q Wave of Infarction

The origin of the Q wave of infarction is diagrammed in Fig. 11-3. Consider two masses of muscle in a volume conductor depolarizing simultaneously over a period of 0.08 s, in opposite directions, and viewed from the positive electrode of a unipolar lead placed so that the thicker mass depolarizes toward it and the thinner away from it (A). During the early phase of the process, the forces balance each other and no deflection is produced; later, depolarization has been completed in the tissue on the left, but continues in that on the right, an unopposed force directed toward the electrode, writing an upstroke. In (B), the shaded area in the larger mass represents dead tissue, capable of transmitting electricity but not generating it. In the early part of depolarization, the only force is directed away from the electrode, writing a negative curve. Later forces, generated in the larger mass after the process has been completed in the smaller one, are directed toward the electrode, producing a final upstroke. Changes in the heart as a result of myocardial infarction are much like these. Wilson described it this way: "a large infarct, which, being composed of dead and inactive muscle, has an effect upon the electrocardiogram similar to that which might be produced by a window or orifice in the anterior wall of the heart."[926]

Location of the Infarct

The most important reason to specify the location of an infarct is for credibility; to report one without saying where evidence for it is seen would be like making a diagnosis of pneumonia without saying which lung is involved. Those seen in precordial leads are commonly classified as anteroseptal or anterolateral, but all this seems to mean is that abnormality is seen in V1–3 or V4–6, not really whether the IV septum is involved; it may be involved with inferior lesions as well as anterior, but this is rarely suggested.[878,879] It is enough to designate the location as simply anterior (seen in precordial leads), lateral (leads I, AVL, II, V6), or inferior (leads II, III, and AVF). Anterior infarcts generally represent lesions in the left anterior descending coronary artery; lateral ones, the circumflex; and inferior ones, the right, but this is not very important, and

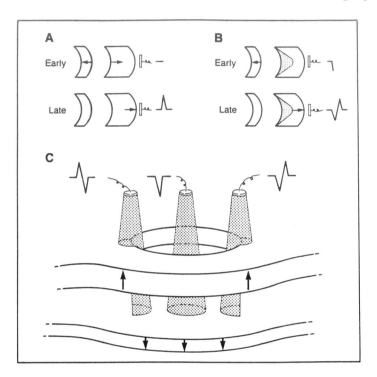

Fig. 11-3. Schematic derivation of the abnormal Q of infarction.

is especially uncertain in differentiating between circumflex and right coronary artery lesions.[871,872] A truly dorsal infarct would be expected to produce an abnormal initial R in V1, but anatomic correlation of findings in electrocardiograms with isolated dorsal infarction is difficult and not well documented[230,231,748,862] (*see* p. 165 for differential diagnosis of prominent RV1). Infarcts are not bounded by straight lines and may be seen from more than one view; e.g., anterolateral, inferodorsal. EKG patterns can be correlated with autopsy findings, but the point whose position the tracing records represents activity in the whole heart, not separate parts of it.

Recognition of infarction of the *right ventricle*[894] is important because of the management it suggests, but it is a clinical entity, not an EKG diagnosis. It is suspected when a patient with an acute inferior infarct and clear lungs has hypotension and jugular venous prominence. Elevation of ST in V4R is supportive evidence.[720,723,731,749–751,858]

When an infarct has been identified by clinical and laboratory means, but there is no abnormality of the initial part of QRS, especially if there is depression of ST in anterior or inferior leads, it is often assumed that the reason it is not visible is that it involves the deep, electrically invisible, or *silent*, part of the myocardium (p. 76), and a diagnosis of *subendocardial* infarction, as distinct from *transmural*, may be made. There may be some clinical value to this differential, but is not an EKG diagnosis.[227,228,266-270,405,674-676,724,725,728-730] The anatomic characteristics of the coronary blood supply dictate that all infarcts, at least generically, are deep, or "subendocardial."

Flattened depression of ST is typical of coronary insufficiency (p. 206), and coronary insufficiency is the means by which an infarct is produced, but an infarct is not identified in the ST-T. To call a lesion transmural when it presents as a QR is not logical; the R must derive from tissue between the infarct and the electrode. A transmural infarct produces a QS pattern in a lead from over its surface:[232] A completely intramural one may be identified in some instances by notches, but only with the aid of special techniques.[5,226,673]

One gets the impression from the literature that the nomenclature is shifting away from *subendocardial* for those that cannot be identified in the EKG, and *transmural* for those that can, to *non-Q-wave* and *Q-wave*. All these labels have limitations, but the newer ones seem more reasonable. To assume that subendocardial, or non-Q-wave, infarcts are limited to the inner layers of the myocardium is to assume that the inner part of the myocardium is indeed electrically invisible, and that, if the EKG were as sensitive to this part as to the outer part, they would be apparent. There is controversy as to whether this "silence" of the "subendocardium" is real, or consistent from individual to individual.[725,728] Certainly there is good evidence that some lesions involving only the deepest layers do produce abnormal Q waves, but the very existence of the terminology attests to the evidence that some do not. At least part of the problem is one of quantitative definition of subendocardium and subepicardium. Anyone who has followed EKGs during cardiac catheterization, and used the exploring needle as a V lead during pericardiocentesis, must have noted the marked difference between the exquisite sensitivity of the tracing to subepicardial injury and the lack of it to subendocardial injury. If *subendocardial* is read as simply deep to subepicardial, and the concept of *electrical endocardium*[927] is accepted, there is no conflict (*see also* p. 77).

    Illogical though it may be, sometimes it is possible at least to suspect an infarct from a QR configuration in a PVC.[272–274]

Age of an Infarct

    An estimate of whether the lesion is old or new is part of the diagnosis of every infarct, and is based on the presence or absence of ST displacement, i.e., evidence of injury (p. 202). It assumes that, because injury is transient, whatever caused it must have occurred recently, and that the critical abnormality early in QRS is explained by the same thing. The typical evidence of recent origin is elevation of ST in leads that show the infarct. Routine lead positions are not such that each is opposite another, and the reverse of this pattern, ST depression, may or may not show, depending on the location of the lesion. ST is often depressed in precordial leads when the infarct is inferior, but less frequently in inferior leads when it is anterior. Presumably this means that with inferior lesions injury forces are directed dorsad as well as caudad, whereas those in most anterior lesions are directed almost entirely ventrad.[773,839,857] ST evidence of injury usually lasts no more than three or four weeks, often very much less, sometimes only minutes or hours, and may not be seen at all. In the absence of the ST-T picture of injury, it is assumed that the lesion is old, but it may not be. Another basis for calling an infarct new is to find evidence of one where there had been none a short time before. Truly transmural infarcts produce little if any ST displacement.[232] Sometimes the ST picture of acute injury may be permanent, and this suggests a ventricular aneurysm (p. 185).

Accuracy of the Diagnosis

    Evaluation of the accuracy of the EKG diagnosis of an infarct depends on correlation with anatomic reality. This requires definitions for both EKG and anatomic findings, and there is less than universal agreement about either. The meaning of infarction is perfectly clear at a conceptual level, but quantitative criteria for the anatomic lesion merge with those for patchy fibrosis, and electro-cardiographic criteria are even more nebulous. Experience teaches that the picture described above, abnormal Q with ST displace-ment, found in a patient with the clinical picture of a "heart attack," is very nearly pathognomonic of a new infarct, and good evidence of an old one is almost as secure,[233–235,441] but there is no way to "rule one out" by EKG. Acute infarction almost always produces some abnormality in the tracing, at least nonspecific ST-T abnor-malities,[904,905] and a normal tracing is strong evidence against the diagnosis, but old lesions often disappear without a trace.[236–239] One report based on autopsy findings implied that as many as 50% of acute infarcts were not recognized in life,[726] but in this study a lesion had to be only 5 mm in its largest diameter to qualify as an infarct. It is probably reasonable to say that about 30% of acute infarcts, as defined by clinical and laboratory methods, are not identifiable in the electrocardiogram.

Summary

The EKG diagnosis of myocardial infarction rests on evidence of two things, an anatomic lesion deep in the wall of the ventricle, and the presence or absence of injury; and two assumptions, that both of these represent the same pathologic process, and that that is inadequacy of blood supply. Other explanations for each of the find-ings are possible, but the combination is so typical that, when the clinical picture suggests an infarct, it is safe to say that the tracing shows one. Absence of evidence, however, is not evidence of absence; to "rule out" an infarct is like trying to "rule out" flying saucers— it can't be done. A normal tracing practically excludes the diagno-sis of a recent one, but not an old one or the presence of extensive coronary atherosclerosis.[240] Stigmata of an infarct may be canceled by a second one,[644,676] or by coronary artery bypass grafting,[626,627] and an old one may leave no identifiable abnormality at all. The finding without which the diagnosis cannot be made is abnormality of initial QRS forces, but that is not either entirely objective or the only thing that counts. Interpretation of a Q wave, for instance, is influenced, not only by the features described above, intrinsic and extrinsic, but also by whether it was there before, and by associated findings, especially the ST-T pattern.

Differential Diagnosis

The EKG abnormalities typical of an infarct identify an anatomic lesion with confidence, but not what caused it; there are explanations for electrical inactivity other than infarction. *False positives* are a real danger because of their prognostic implication, and they may be produced in many ways. First, of course, the limits of the method; normal findings are not always neatly separable from abnormal ones. It is not a Q wave that is the hallmark of an infarct, but abnormality of the initial part of the QRS. This usually means an abnormal Q, but definition of *abnormal* is not precise (p. 174). Qs that could easily be called abnormal may be seen even in healthy young people,[258,259] and, in the absence of control tracings, can introduce a problem when these people present with vague substernal or epigastric discomfort, when they seek employment or permission to engage in athletics, or when they are qualifying for insurance.

Noncardiac disorders may produce EKG findings that simulate those of an infarct. Pectus excavatum, and the straight back syndrome,[242,243] and hyperkalemia[249,516] for instance, as well as pulmonary disease, especially embolism, cor pulmonale,[614] and pneumothorax.[251,493,615,772] Pancreatitis is often mentioned in the literature as capable of producing similar findings,[241] but this is probably not true;[864] ST-T abnormalities, yes, but QRS abnormalities, no. Precordial Q waves may be rate dependent.[665]

Diseases of the heart other than infarction may explain many false positives. There are not many congenital lesions in this category, but subendocardial fibroelastosis and corrected transposition of the great vessels have been reported as doing it.[247,629] Ventricular pre-excitation (the Wolff–Parkinson–White Syndrome) is a common offender,[189,191,618] and scarring may be part of idiopathic cardiac myopathy,[244–246] sarcoid,[619] amyloid, muscular dystrophy,[620] or infectious mononucleosis.[617] Asymmetric septal hypertrophy, or idiopathic hypertrophic subaortic stenosis, may change the initial part of the QRS as a result of enlarging the mass of the IV septum,[452,727] left ventricular hypertrophy alone may do the same thing,[256,257,721] and so can right ventricular enlargement.[722] Left anterior hemiblock has been reported as mimicking myocardial infarction,[440,511,538,621,622,691] and so has mitral valve prolapse.[502] Dorsal infarction may be simulated by abnormally directed anterior forces resulting from block of a septal segment of the intraventricular conduction system (p. 165).[623,699] Right atrial enlargement may be a big factor in abnormality of the Q,[8,248] pericardial effusion has been found as the explanation for EKG findings of infarction,[624] and abnormalities caused by cardiac surgery[250] or blunt trauma[252,616] are easy to understand. Similar findings may be produced by artificial ventricular pacemakers,[482,677] and the first part of the QRS may be distorted by merging with P as in isorhythmic dissociation or atrial flutter.

Technical error can produce EKG findings that mimic infarction, most commonly transposition of left arm and leg leads, right arm and leg leads, occasionally right and left arm leads, and inappropriate positioning of electrodes for precordial leads, e.g., transposition of V1 and V3 (p. 109). Individual leads mounted upside down can produce a problem, and other errors are possible.[253,255]

There may be *false negatives*, too, but they introduce less risk; failure to recognize an infarct from the EKG alone is not likely to hurt the patient; the doctor who ordered the study knows the clinical setting, and there are other ways to make the diagnosis. Evidence of an infarct may be obscured by an idioventricular pacemaker, an artificial ventricular pacemaker, ventricular pre-excitation, left bundle branch block (pp. 161, 170), errors of lead placement, especially swapping of the left arm and left leg leads, and such unusual events as pneumothorax.[772]

The manifestations of infarction may be transient,[260–263,759] disappearing following coronary artery bypass,[626,627] as a result of cancellation of potentials when the tissue opposite an infarct is infarcted itself,[644,676] or for no identifiable reason.

There is every reason to believe that infarcts do occur without being suspected clinically, and that these might be identifiable in the electrocardiogram, *silent* infarcts,[625,725,726] but proof of this is difficult, and to assume that EKG findings suggestive, even typical, of an infarct are proof that there has been one, even though there is no clinical support for it, is not justified. To accept a computer readout alone is inappropriate.

Miscellaneous

A diagnosis of *left anterior fascicular block* in the presence of an inferior infarct is probably inappropriate. Either may cause left axis deviation, and they may coexist, but identification of both in a single tracing is outside the limits of the method. This problem is discussed on p. 164.

Some QRS widening is common with myocardial infarction and is not satisfactorily explained. The concept of *peri-infarction block* (p. 168) has been proposed for a long time as an explanation for not only this but also changes in the terminal part of QRS.

Signal averaging methods developed in recent years have made it possible to identify small, high-frequency signals related to depolarization. These are called *late potentials* or *after depolarizations* and are designated as *early* when they occur near the junction of QRS and ST, and *late* when they coincide with the U wave. They are thought to be related to some kind of re-entrant "triggering" of ventricular ectopy, and the early ones, when found in a patient recovering from a myocardial infarct, have been shown to have predictive value for later occurrence of ventricular fibrillation, especially of the *torsades de pointes* variety (p. 146). The late ones may help explain acquired prolonged QT-U syndromes (p. 234), not only the electrocardiographic picture but also the propensity to ventricular fibrillation.[895,929,936]

The *time necessary for appearance* of EKG changes of infarction is hard to specify. How long does it take for the anatomic change, without which EKG evidence cannot be validated, to develop? How is the exact time at which the critical events took place to be defined? Observations following accidental occlusion of coronary arteries at surgery or arteriography have led to the impression that, though ST-T abnormalities of coronary insufficiency may appear almost immediately, the QRS change of infarction may take as long as twelve hours, and there is some experimental evidence to support this.[413,754] Sometimes it does not appear at all.

The *number of infarcts* that can be diagnosed from a single tracing is, strictly speaking, not more than one; evidence in two views does not necessarily mean two infarcts. Because of the anatomy of the coronary blood supply, and the position of the leads with relation to the heart, both anterior and inferior lesions, and sometimes lateral ones, can be diagnosed with confidence either in serial tracings or the same one, but real proof of multiple infarcts depends upon information other than that in the tracing.[275] Quantitative factors come into play; how many cells have to be lost to distinguish an episode of angina from an infarct?

Complications of myocardial infarction recognized in the EKG are mostly disorders of impulse formation and conduction, "electrical failure."[145,276–278] An unusual complication is *ventricular aneurysm*, and this may be suspected when ST displacement persists more than a few days following an acute infarct. The explanation for this is not clear, but it must represent some continuing impairment of electrophysiologic function in the tissue immediately surrounding the aneurysm.[223,279,414,755,775,843]

The atria are subject to infarction just as the ventricles are, but *atrial infarcts* are not often diagnosed. They show mostly in the PQ segment, and recognition requires compromise in definition of the baseline (p. 9). The diagnosis is tenuous at best.[280–282,395,645,756–758]

TWELVE

Atrial and Ventricular Enlargement

The third major application of electrocardiography, after analysis of impulse formation and conduction, and the differential diagnosis of chest pain, is for recognition of hemodynamic lesions. Here, as elsewhere, the nomenclature is inconsistent, and quantitative standards for even such basic concepts as *enlargement*, *dilatation*, *hypertrophy*, and *strain* are not always agreed on. Nevertheless, it is often possible to point to one or more chambers as the seat of disproportionate hemodynamic burden.

Some definitions are in order. In this discussion, *load* refers to the amount of work a chamber is required to perform in order to keep the blood moving forward; *overload* and *strain* are used as synonyms to imply a load greater than normal. The anatomic result of overload is hypertrophy and/or dilatation. *Hypertrophy* means increase in muscle mass; *dilatation*, increase in the volume of a chamber, and, when distinction between them is not clear, the word is *enlargement*. There is a difference between strain (function) and enlargement (structure), and this difference can often be detected electrocardiographically. Just as weight lifters' muscles hurt long before their biceps bulge, EKG evidence of strain typically precedes that of hypertrophy.

Atrial Enlargement

Atrial repolarization is not defined well enough in the tracing to permit recognition of atrial strain, but it is possible to suspect enlargement of one or both chambers from the size and shape of P. The atria depolarize sequentially, right before left (p. 75); events originating in the right are seen best in the frontal plane, while those in the left show better in V1.

187

Right Atrial Enlargement

Right atrial enlargement causes prominence of P in leads II, III, and AVF ("P pulmonale") (Fig. 12-1) and, less consistently, the initial, positive component of P in V1. It may also explain prominence of Q in V1 in the absence of a myocardial infarct.[248,285,286,289,763] (Fig. 12-1). Prominence, though, is in the eye of the beholder, not something for which precise criteria can be specified. Amplitude, contour, duration, area, and the relation of all of these to QRS and to previous tracings and the interpreter's experience, are factors. Perhaps the contour, tented or peaked, and area and amplitude, large with relation to QRS, are most important.

Left Atrial Enlargement

Left atrial enlargement is recognized by prominence of the terminal part of P in V1, i.e., width and depth each at least one millimeter (Fig. 12-2).[287-290,764,938] It may produce exaggerated notching of P, and some widening, especially in lead II, but a small notch is a normal characteristic of P waves.

Miscellaneous

The ratio of the duration of the P wave to the PR segment, the Macruz index, was proposed as a means of recognizing atrial enlargement but is not very useful.[291] Peaking of P in Lead I has been called *P congenitale*.[928]

Discussion

Aside from rare familial and idiopathic instances, overload is the only explanation for enlargement of a chamber, and overload can result from one, or both, of only two things, increase in the volume of blood the chamber is called upon to pump per unit of time, or in the force opposing it, flow and resistance. Left atrial enlargement represents response to mitral regurgitation or stenosis, left ventricular failure, or loss of compliance of the left ventricle; right atrial enlargement, comparable abnormalities of the tricuspid valve and right ventricle. The electrocardiogram is very sensitive to right atrial enlargement,

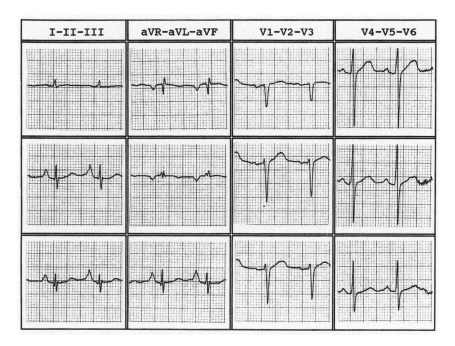

Fig. 12-1. Right atrial enlargement.

and this is often the first, or only, evidence in the tracing of loss of compliance by the right ventricle, especially common in patients whose primary lesion is in the lungs. Enlargement of either atrium may be transient, waxing or waning within hours, or even minutes, as with response to treatment or during exercise testing, suggesting that dilatation is probably the principal change rather than hypertrophy. The increase in flow resulting from an atrial septal defect imposes an additional burden on the left atrium, but little EKG change.[946]

Ventricular Strain

Change in the EKG in response to overload of a ventricle would be expected to appear first in the most sensitive part of the ventricular complex, the T wave, and this happens very often. The change is not specific, of course—T abnormality is never specific—but, in

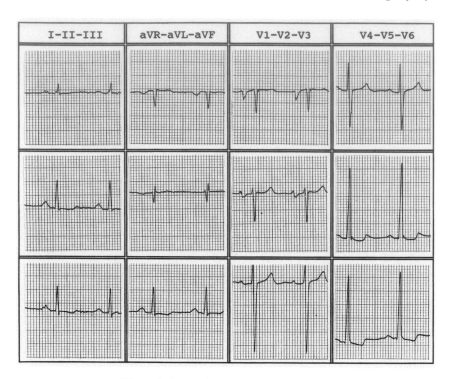

Fig. 12-2. Left atrial enlargement.

the case of the left ventricle, commonly takes a form characteristic enough to be suggestive; an otherwise normal T directed nearly opposite QRS, i.e., negative in leads with positive QRSs, usually I and V6, but with normal duration, amplitude, and contour (Fig. 12-3). J may be depressed in the same leads, but ST is not flattened; and J depression in this setting, with normal ST contour and normal or exaggerated T voltage, probably represents the same events called "early repolarization" when ST is elevated in the same leads (p. 205).

This pattern presumably reflects changes deep in the ventricular myocardium that result from the increased vigor of contraction in response to overload, and these undoubtedly include at least some lessening of the reserve supply of blood (oxygen) available. When the reserve is adequate, this is not critical, but when it is diminished, and/or the increase in demand is excessive, change in physiology is induced. If this explanation is right, the discrepancy it

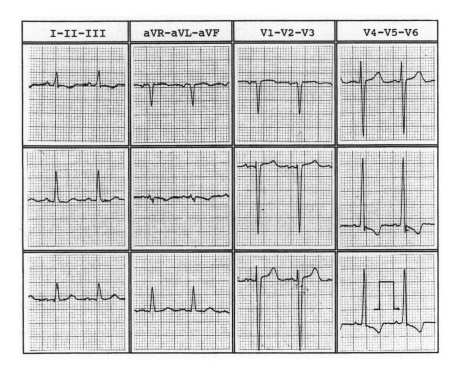

| I–II–III | aVR–aVL–aVF | V1–V2–V3 | V4–V5–V6 |

Fig. 12-3. Left ventricular overload (strain).

represents could be brought about by diminution of supply just as logically as by increase in demand, and both may be involved at the same time. The clinical setting and stability of the findings are important in the differential. If there is QRS evidence of left ventricular hypertrophy, for instance, the ST-T pattern is stable, and the patient is hypertensive, the probability that it represents left ventricular strain is strengthened; if QRS is normal, the ST-T abnormality transient, and the problem is substernal pain, coronary insufficiency is more likely, but, given only the ST-T abnormality, a single tracing, and no knowledge of the clinical circumstances, left ventricular overload is the first choice. The patterns more likely to represent coronary insufficiency are discussed on pp. 206 and 211.

It would be just as logical to speak of right ventricular strain as left, but the vocabulary for the right ventricle is different from that of the left. How this came to be is not clear, but it may be logical.

Dilatation is probably a bigger factor in determining the EKG picture of overload of the right ventricle than of the left, and physiologic change in the relatively massive wall of the left ventricle has a greater influence on the tracing than in the thin one of the right. Negative T waves in right precordial leads sometimes do correlate with overload of the right ventricle, as with pulmonary embolism, but are common in normals, especially children and young adults (p. 236).

Ventricular Hypertrophy

Depolarization of a large mass of muscle generates greater voltage and produces a larger deflection than depolarization of a small mass; hypertrophy of one ventricle, not balanced by equal hypertrophy of the other, would be expected to direct the QRS more counterclockwise and posteriorly in the case of the left ventricle, and clockwise and anteriorly in the case of the right. This does occur, but the range of normal for QRS orientation is so wide, and change can be brought about by so many things (p. 226), that QRS axis alone is not very helpful as a marker of ventricular enlargement.

It seems reasonable, too, to assume that the time required for activation of the ventricular wall from endocardium to epicardium, the *ventricular activation time* (VAT), would correlate with the thickness of the wall.[939] This appealing idea has received a lot of attention, but has two limitations; depolarization is not a simple straight-line process, and, probably even more important, estimation of the *time* from the beginning of QRS to the intrinsic, or *intrinsicoid*, deflection, the peak of R, is not practical. In the normal adult it is said to be not more than 0.04 s in a left chest lead, and 0.02 s in one from the right, greater values suggesting hypertrophy of the left or right ventricle, but routine tracings cannot be measured this closely.

Left Ventricular Hypertrophy

The only EKG finding that has much value as evidence of *left ventricular hypertrophy* is QRS amplitude (voltage), and that is influenced by many factors besides the mass of ventricular muscle. The distance of the electrodes from the heart, the conductivity of intervening tissues, the volume and temperature of blood in the ventricles, the recording equipment, and other features less easily identifiable must all be taken into account (p. 228); nonetheless, high QRS voltage does suggest left ventricular hypertrophy. Sokolow and Lyon's criterion,[293] the sum of SV1 and RV5 (or RV6, whichever is taller) greater than 3.5 mV, is probably the one most widely used, identifying it in something over 80% of cases.[294] Voltage may vary widely from day to day, though, even from beat to beat, and to call this figure closer than 0.5 mV is not practical. A value of 4.0 is not clearly abnormal; 4.5 must be taken seriously but still is not enough by itself to make a diagnosis of left ventricular hypertrophy. At 5.0 mV left ventricular hypertrophy must be considered likely (Fig. 12-4). Hypertrophy and strain can often be suspected in the same tracing (Fig. 12-5).

Right Ventricular Enlargement

Right ventricular enlargement produces two typical patterns, and in thinking about them it is helpful to be aware that, though the right ventricle is to the right of the left border of the heart in the frontal projection, it is wholly anterior; the right border of the cardiac silhouette is made up of the venae cavae and right atrium, not right ventricle. Dilatation is suspected when the frontal axis is indeterminate and the precordial QRS transition zone is broad (Fig. 12-6), often with an rSr in V1 and a prominent S in V6, a pattern seen especially with flow lesions, diastolic overload, as with atrial septal defect. Hypertrophy can be diagnosed with confidence when there is a tall R in V1 and a deep S in V6 (Fig. 12-7), a pattern typical of systolic overload of the right ventricle, as with pulmonary stenosis. Findings less clear-cut than these may be normal or reflect response of the right ventricle to pulmonary disease or other overload.[295,296] Evidence of right atrial enlargement in the same tracing strengthens the diagnosis of right ventricular enlargement, and is especially helpful when QRS evidence is equivocal.

Discussion

It seems reasonable to expect the early, functional manifestations of strain of a ventricle to be apparent before evidence of structural response occurs, and evidence of hypertrophy without strain

I–II–III	aVR–aVL–aVF	V1–V2–V3	V4–V5–V6

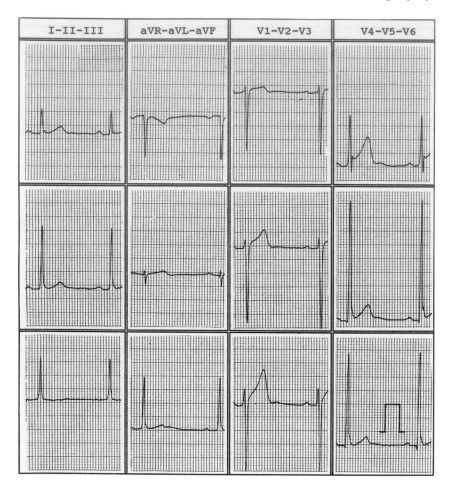

Fig. 12-4. Left ventricular hypertrophy.

to be found when physiologic change is proportional to overload, and these separate patterns do occur, but their specificity is limited. The one typical of strain probably represents discrepancy between supply and demand for blood, and can be produced by restriction of blood supply as easily as by overload of the ventricle. Given serial tracings to establish the transient nature of the findings or their stability, this picture can be useful, at least as corroborative evidence in either case when the clinical setting is known, but by itself it is more likely to represent hemodynamic burden on the ventricle.

I-II-III	aVR-aVL-aVF	V1-V2-V3	V4-V5-V6

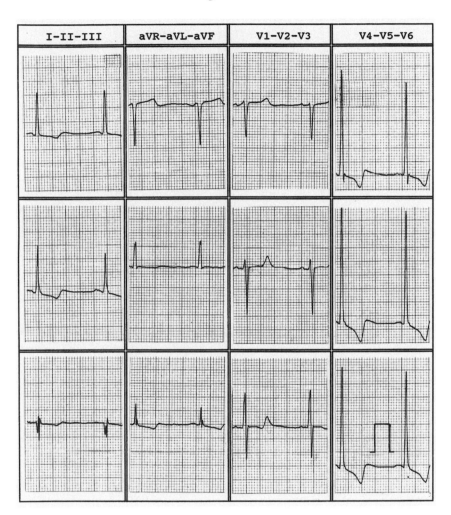

Fig. 12-5. Left ventricular hypertrophy and strain.

Ockham's razor being what it is, evidence of hypertrophy in the same tracing increases the probability that the ST-T pattern means overload.

Hypertrophy of muscle is defined traditionally as increase in the size of cells; increase in their number is *hyperplasia*. Hyperplasia has been shown to occur in the newborn,[547] but is not an important clinical problem. Hypertrophy may be familial, or idiopathic, and

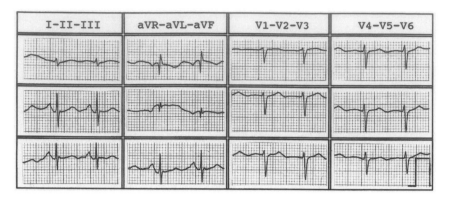

| I–II–III | aVR–aVL–aVF | V1–V2–V3 | V4–V5–V6 |

Fig. 12-6. Right ventricular enlargement, probably dilatation.

hypoxia may be a factor,[579] but is almost always a response to a load beyond what can be accommodated comfortably. Despite the clear meaning of the words *hypertrophy, dilatation,* and *strain,* usage has blurred the distinction among them;[861,863] radiologists often report left ventricular hypertrophy, for instance, when what they see is probably mostly dilatation. Echocardiography has not been very helpful,[605] and, clear as the concept of strain is, proof of it, other than demonstration of a lesion that would necessitate it, is problematic.

How, then, is the EKG evidence suggesting either hypertrophy or strain to be evaluated? With what can the findings be correlated? The answer is lesions that overload one ventricle or the other selectively. This has the advantage of being simple, easy, not requiring autopsy, and what we are really interested in anyway. Sokolow and Lyon's numbers, even though they are used as evidence of hypertrophy,[293] were validated this way, as were those in a recent large European study.[937]

Overload of the left ventricle is a consequence of either one or both of only two possibilities: increase in flow, and increase in resistance. Flow lesions that overload the left ventricle (and not the right) are valve regurgitation (aortic and mitral) and shunts (ventricular septal defect and ductus arteriosus); increase in resistance may reside in the peripheral arterioles (hypertension, especially diastolic), larger arteries (hypertension, especially systolic),

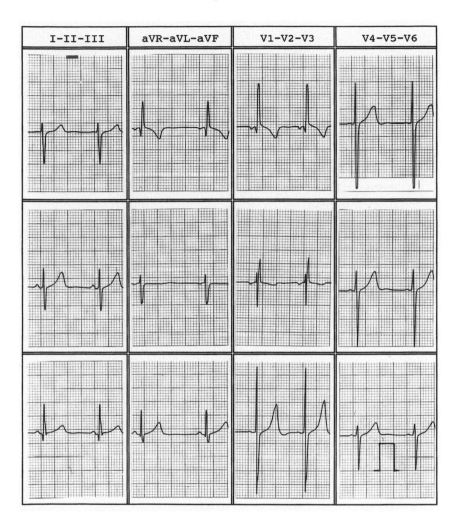

Fig. 12-7. Right ventricular hypertrophy.

aorta (coarctation), and/or the outflow tract (where obstruction may be supravalvular, valvular, or subvalvular). That's all, and each of these can be identified easily by physical examination. The same observations can be applied to lesions that overload the right ventricle. Increase in blood viscosity affects both ventricles, and so do peripheral AV shunts.

Miscellaneous

The electrocardiographic definition of *biventricular hypertrophy* is a tenuous thing indeed, based on little logic. Equal hypertrophy of both ventricles would be expected to result in either large complexes or no change. It is unlikely that hypertrophy is ever confined strictly to one ventricle; there is no clear anatomic dividing line between them, and metabolic changes affecting one must affect the other to some extent also. Nonetheless, clinical experience leaves the impression that, when the picture of left ventricular overload is seen inferiorly (leads II, III, and F) better than laterally, and there are strong anterior forces and/or evidence of right atrial enlargement, a suspicion of biventricular hypertrophy is justified.[298]

Bundle branch block and ventricular hypertrophy may coexist, of course, but diagnosis of both from a single tracing is not logical; the presence of an intraventricular conduction defect means that the ventricles are not being depolarized simultaneously, and the numbers used as evidence of hypertrophy were acquired from subjects with normal intraventricular conduction. Both hypertrophy and bundle branch block serve to direct attention to the named ventricle, but hypertrophy (or strain, enlargement, or overload) is a response by the ventricle to a burden imposed from outside, while bundle branch block identifies a lesion in the ventricular wall. Sometimes distinction between hypertrophy and bundle branch block is arbitrary.[209–211,299–301,442,765,886] Lesions that overload a ventricle may precipitate bundle branch block, but not vice versa.

Summary

Right atrial enlargement is recognized by prominence and symmetry of P in leads II, III, and aVF; left, by prominence of the terminally negative component of P in V1.

If the sum of the amplitude of SV1 and RV5 (or RV6, whichever is taller) is large, in the absence of another explanation for high voltage, left ventricular hypertrophy must be suspected; if the QRS is directed to the left while the T is directed nearly opposite, left ventricular strain. When the QRS is directed anteriorly, or is nearly biphasic in all leads, right ventricular hypertrophy, or at least enlargement, is suspected. Evidence of atrial enlargement is indirect support for a suspicion of ventricular enlargement.

The diagnosis of ventricular overload, by whatever name, should have only one specific effect, to insure that the possibility of a disproportionate hemodynamic burden seen by that ventricle is considered. Ventricular hypertrophy is not a disease itself but a response to disease. Failure to recognize it in the tracing is not likely to hurt a patient who has had a history and physical examination, but to suggest it from the tracing alone may produce harm if the limitations of the method are not recognized.

THIRTEEN

Abnormalities of Ventricular Repolarization

The specificity–sensitivity spectrum of the ventricular complex can be compared to a pennant on a pole (Fig. 2-9, p. 44); even the smallest breeze can move the tip, a stronger wind will straighten it out all the way, and a real hurricane will bend the pole. When the wind subsides, the pennant will return to its undisturbed position, alongside the pole if the pole is still vertical, but apart from it if the pole has been bent. QRS-ST-T abnormalities are similar in many respects. Change may be induced in T by almost any stimulus, even a drink of cold water, a more severe or sustained one is needed to affect the ST segment, and QRS abnormality, especially of duration or contour, almost always means structural abnormality in the ventricular wall. T and ST may return to normal when the stimulus is removed, but QRS abnormality is likely to persist. Change in the route of depolarization influences that of repolarization; abnormality in ST-T may be secondary to that in QRS.

QRS abnormalities, and their reflection in ST-T, have been discussed in preceding chapters; this one is concerned mostly with primary, intrinsic ST-T patterns as evidence of abnormality of function not affecting structure. Describing and naming these is more difficult than with P or QRS, because ST-T is a continuous line, and change in one part affects the other as well. The asymmetric nature of the curve, though, makes it possible to distinguish between a proximal part in which the slope is very gentle, the ST segment, and a distal, steeper one, the T.

The orientation, amplitude, and contour of these subdivisions can be described separately to a large extent, but repolarization begins while depolarization is in progress, and the only option for considering its *duration* is to treat it as beginning at the same point as QRS. With this as a given, the length of QT is a function of where T ends, and it takes very little experience to realize that this is a rough estimate at best, ideally requiring simultaneous recording of several leads or, at least, averaging of data,[818,942] and the advantage gained by such tedious methods is almost nil. At a clinical level, estimation by inspection is adequate, and 0.04 s is about as close as it can be called meaningfully (p. 23).

QT may be shortened by digitalis, hypercalcemia, increased intracranial pressure,[943] and perhaps other things, but shortening is hard to define, and not likely to be a critical finding; change is almost always prolongation, and prolongation of QT, by itself, is a nonspecific finding (*see* p. 234 for discussion of the long QT syndromes).

The ST Segment

The ST segment has two separate and distinct elements, position and contour, a point and a line, and these must be considered separately. Its *orientation*, displacement or lack of displacement, is defined by the position of the J point with relation to the baseline, at it, above it, or below it in *specified leads*; the *amplitude* of displacement, by how far above or below. Displacement can be determined by the beginner as easily as by anyone, but whether it is abnormal is another question, and the answer depends largely on its *contour*. When abnormal, ST displacement can be translated almost directly to mean myocardial injury, and *injury* is a word whose meaning is exactly the same in electrocardiography as it is in English; it implies impairment of function, and, by its very nature, is transient; injured tissue either gets well or dies. Before criteria for abnormality can be discussed, though, other characteristics of its chief marker, displacement itself, must be considered.

The view from which injury is seen, anterior, inferior, or lateral, is part of the description, but its location in the thickness of the ventricular wall, superficial or deep, *subepicardial* or *subendocardial*, is more important. This can be recognized easily in most instances, and the basis for it can be diagrammed as an application of the principals discussed on p. 78 (Figs. 13-1 and 13-2).

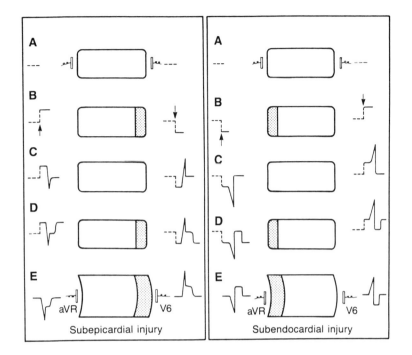

Fig. 13-1 *(left)* and Fig. 13-2 *(right)*. Figure 13-1 shows diagrammatic explanation of ST displacement of subepicardial injury. Figure 13-2 shows an ST displacement of subendocardial injury *(see below)*.

From an electrophysiologic point of view, injury can be defined as inability of the damaged myocardium to be polarized completely, to hold a charge. Figure 13-1(A) shows a resting muscle strip in a volume conductor viewed from the exploring electrodes of two unipolar leads, one at each end. The tissue is polarized. There is a difference in potential between the inside of the strip and the outside, but this is not apparent to a galvanometer that sees only the outside, and when the paper is drawn past the stylus a flat line is written (dotted). In (B) the shaded area on the right represents injury. Injured tissue is not completely polarized, but the adjacent normal tissue is, and, at the onset of injury (arrow), a boundary of potential difference exists between the two. The electrode at the left faces the

positive side of this boundary, and the trace recorded from it registers this by assuming a position above the baseline; that on the
right, its negative side, and the trace is deflected downward.

In (C) the injured strip has been depolarized from left to right,
producing an upstroke in the tracing on the right and a downstroke
in the one on the left (*see* Fig. 2-6, p. 33); injury does not interfere
with depolarization, and when this process has been completed there
is no difference of potential in the system, and the trace returns to
the level that indicates this, true zero, the level of the dotted line in
(A). In (D), repolarization has occurred, re-establishing a potential
difference between normal and injured tissue, and the trace resumes
the level that is a measure of this, producing elevation of ST from
one view and depression from the other.

An alternative interpretation of these events is to see them as
shifting the baseline, not the ST, but this is in conflict with the
definition of a baseline as establishing a fixed level for reference,
and ignores the fact that injury produces change in ventricular repolarization, represented by ST-T, not PR. Baselines do not change,
and the definition on p. 9 is still valid.

Figure 13-1(E) shows schematically how similar these examples
are to the situation that exists when a layer of muscle beneath the
epicardium of the left ventricle is injured. The electrode at the left
may be compared to AVR and that at the right to V6. There is
elevation of ST in the lead that sees the outside of the heart (V6),
and depression on the opposite side. This is typical of superficial,
or *subepicardial*, injury, as seen with inflammation of the pericardium.
Figure 13-2 shows the same series of events except that the injured
tissue is at the left end of the muscle strip, comparable to the deep,
or *subendocardial*, layers of the ventricular myocardium where
injury is usually related to coronary insufficiency. Note that in each
case the tracing as a whole shows ST displacement, up in some
leads and down in others, different views of the same thing, not two
things, one "reciprocal" to the other (Fig. 13-3).

Now consider these events as expressed in an electrocardiogram, their description and interpretation. Decisions about whether
ST displacement is abnormal depends on its magnitude, contour,
and stability, and stability cannot be assessed from a single tracing.

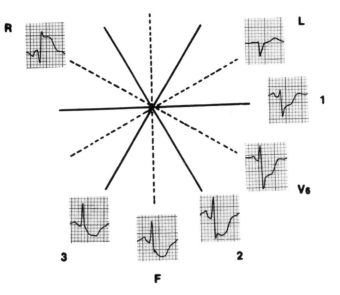

Fig. 13-3. ST displacement away from one point is toward another. There is only one ST; the tracing shows twelve views of it.

First, *displacement*. The rate at which energy is stored during repolarization varies. In some hearts, the amount generated while QRS is being written is so small that it does not show at all, and the trace is at the baseline at the end of QRS. In many normal hearts, though, the process is more vigorous; the trace is well on its way toward writing T when QRS ends, and J is clearly apart from the baseline. This is especially common in right precordial leads where ST is elevated, often a millimeter or more, and, when the contour is normal *(see below)*, this calls for no comment. It is common in leads from the left side, too, especially when QRS and T are both tall, and still normal, but here it rates a name, *early repolarization* (Fig. 13-4), and it may be difficult to distinguish between this pattern and the one so typical of subepicardial injury, especially when there is only one tracing and the clinical problem is not known. The more marked the displacement (in proportion to QRS amplitude), and the flatter the contour *(see below)*, the more likely it is to be abnormal. If an earlier tracing is not available for control, a later

I–II–III	aVR–aVL–aVF	V1–V2–V3	V4–V5–V6

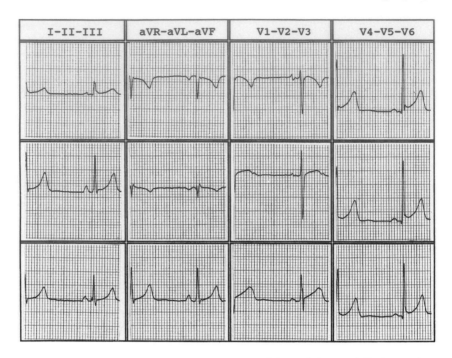

Fig. 13-4. Description of abnormalities of ST and T (*see also* Fig. 2-10).

one may serve the same purpose; "early repolarization" is normal and the pattern will not change, but injury is transient.[223,224,510,512,553,669] The clinical setting, of course, is crucial.

Displacement can be indicated quantitatively, but *contour* calls for adjectives. The normal ST-T contour, in a lead in which QRS and T are of the same sign, can be described as departing from the baseline at an increasingly rapid rate until maximal amplitude is reached near its distal end, and returning swiftly to the baseline, or very near it. Abnormality of the proximal part of this line, ST, can be indicated by such adjectives as sagging (describing a catenary curve), flattened (horizontal), arched (the reverse of sagging), or straightened (Figs. 2-10, 13-5).

Flattened depression of ST in leads in which QRS is positive or biphasic is typical of *subendocardial, or deep, injury* (Fig. 13-6). It

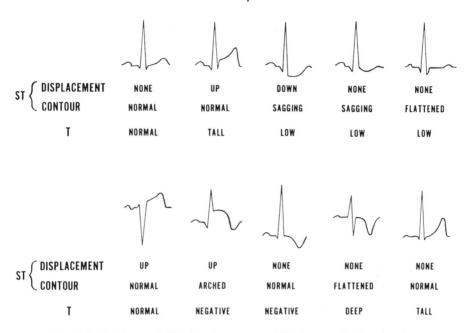

Fig. 13-5. Normal ST displacement. "Early repolarization."

might be expected that this could be produced by a catheter, a pacemaker electrode, or a wayward central venous pressure line, but it is not seen in these settings, probably because of the lesser electrical sensitivity of the inner layers of the ventricular myocardium (p. 76). The most frequent explanation for it is the obvious one; the tissue in question is at the distal end of the arterial system, the area most sensitive to impairment of blood flow. When it is transient, and the clinical picture suggests coronary insufficiency, flattened depression of ST is almost pathognomonic. Coronary insufficiency, though, is not necessarily the same as angina pectoris, and, when there is only one tracing and the clinical setting is not known, other explanations must be considered.

The pattern may be stable and asymptomatic in older people,[672] even in young ones, with no other reason to suspect heart disease, and it has been found frequently during prolonged ambulatory monitoring in the absence of symptoms.[837,838] It may be found in

I-II-III	aVR-aVL-aVF	V1-V2-V3	V4-V5-V6

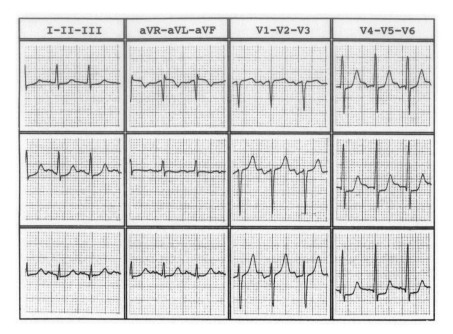

Fig. 13-6. Subendocardial injury, as with coronary insufficiency.

patients with intracranial disease (p. 233), and may result from overdamping of the stylus (p. 98). To equate ST depression with ischemia (p. 136), and ischemia with coronary insufficiency, is a potentially dangerous oversimplification.[954] The significance to the patient of the EKG picture depends on which factors contributed to it, and this is not apparent in the tracing alone.

The sensitivity of the myocardium increases from endocardium toward epicardium, and anything that damages even the most superficial cells is likely to produce an ST response.[225,228,883] *Subepicardial, or superficial, injury* (Fig. 13-7) is usually secondary to inflammation of the pericardium (infection, trauma, neoplasia, or other), but another explanation is outward extension of deep injury. When coronary blood flow is impaired, the tissue affected first is deep, and ST is depressed in most leads, but, as the degree of impairment increases, the injured area extends proximad to involve ever more superficial layers of myocardium, and may be expressed ultimately as ST elevation; the

I-II-III	aVR-aVL-aVF	V1-V2-V3	V4-V5-V6

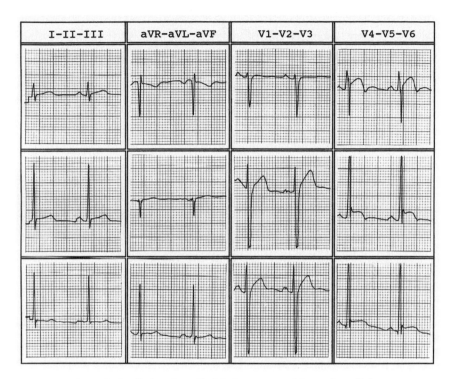

Fig. 13-7. Subepicardial injury, as with pericarditis.

trace cannot be up and down at the same time in the same lead. This is probably the explanation of ST elevation with acute myocardial infarction[529,578,668,769] and may apply also to a similar picture in response to exercise, and in Prinzmetal's, or "variant," angina.[770,771]

ST displacement is usually transient but may persist indefinitely. When it persists following myocardial infarction, it suggests a ventricular aneurysm (p. 185), and the same pattern has been described in patients with asymmetric septal hypertrophy.[768] Leads are not deployed in an equal and opposite fashion, and ST displacement is often seen as only elevation or depression, but when both sides of the picture do show elevation in some leads and depression in others (Fig. 13-3), there is some risk that they may be interpreted as evidence of two lesions instead of two views of the same one.[773,839,857]

In practice, tracings are often said simply to show ST elevation or depression, and this can be interpreted almost always to mean *concordant* displacement, i.e., in the same direction as the net QRS, or *discordant*, opposite QRS. *Elevation* is often used loosely to imply subepicardial injury; *depression*, subendocardial.

Abnormality of contour may be the only abnormality in the tracing, and, when this is the case, its significance is nonspecific, intermediate between abnormality of QRS and abnormality of T.

The T Wave

Abnormality of T, the distal end of the repolarization complex selectively, the most sensitive and least specific part of the tracing, may be primary and/or secondary. The same four measurements applied to other parts of the tracing are applicable, but it is even more difficult to consider them separately here than in the more stable portions.

The *orientation* of T (p. 48) is normal or abnormal only as it relates to QRS. The relation between them, the ventricular gradient, can be compared to that between height and weight, with QRS representing height, the stable component (p. 51). Normally, they are close together in space, not more than about 45° apart in the frontal plane and 60° in the horizontal.

Amplitude and *contour* are inextricably interrelated in further description. Amplitude, voltage, is easy to measure but difficult to assess. Low voltage is the most common and least specific abnormality of T, but just how low it must be to be abnormal is a function of its relation to QRS rather than an absolute figure. A good reference value is that in a lead in which the QRS is almost completely unidirectional, often Lead I or V6, the amplitude of T should be at least 10% of that of QRS. High voltage is even more difficult to define, but 50% of QRS, in leads in which QRS and T are both of the same sign, is as good a figure as any. When voltage is low, contour is rarely mentioned. When it is high, amplitude may be combined with contour, describing T as tall and peaked, or deep and symmetrical.

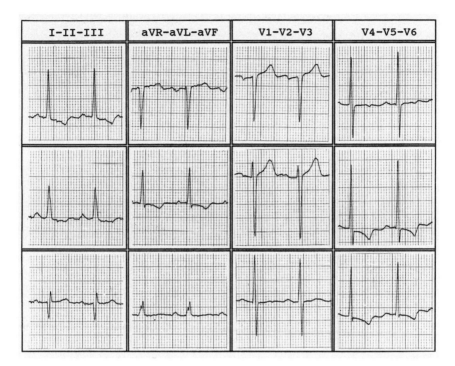

Fig. 13-8. The T wave pattern of left ventricular overload, or strain.

T abnormalities are never specific, but frequently fall into *patterns* that at least suggest one explanation or another. When the spatial angle between QRS and T approximates 180°, and the ST-T contour remains normal, the most likely explanation is *left ventricular overload* (Fig. 13-8) (p. 189), and if there is QRS evidence of left ventricular hypertrophy, something that is almost always a result of overload, the probability that the T pattern means left ventricular overload is enhanced.

Another common pattern expressed mostly in T involves orientation as well as amplitude and contour, and is strong evidence for *coronary insufficiency*. In this picture, T is more nearly symmetrical than usual, deeper in leads from the mid-precordium than in those farther to the right or left (Fig. 13-9), and ST is likely to be arched. When transient and associated with chest pain, this mid-

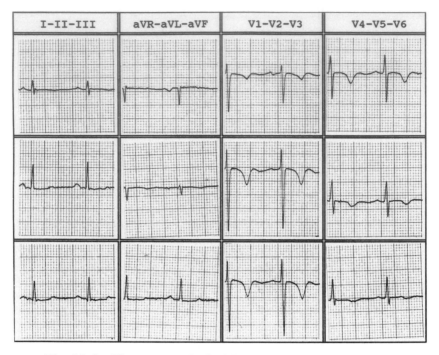

Fig. 13-9. The symmetrical mid-precordial T pattern of coronary insufficiency.

precordial T negativity is almost as secure evidence of coronary insufficiency as flattened depression of ST.

A similar symmetrical T pattern in leads I, II, and III was described in the early 1920s by Pardee and came to be called a *Pardee T wave.* As with all T abnormalities, this one is not specific. Anemia, as in sickle cell crisis, may be a factor, and so may asymmetric septal hypertrophy.[697] The same pattern may be seen in normal children[466] and in healthy young athletes[554] as well as with pheochromocytoma,[643] in patients with hyperparathyroidism,[681] subarachnoid hemorrhage,[503] and concussion.[595] A similar picture with opposite sign, tall, peaked midprecordial T, may represent the same thing.[220,221] Patterns suggestive of both left ventricular overload and coronary insufficiency often may be recognized in the same tracing (Fig. 13-10).

Tall peaked precordial Ts (Fig. 13-11) are common in normals but may be one of the stigmata of hyperkalemia (p. 231), an intra-

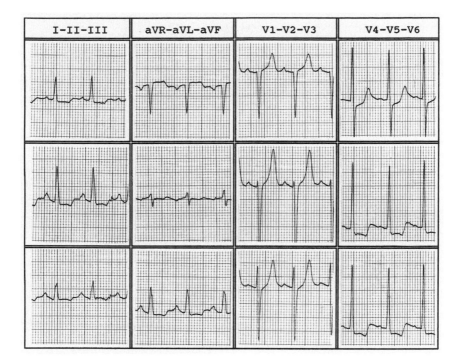

Fig. 13-10. An ST-T pattern suggesting both left ventricular overload and coronary insufficiency.

cranial lesion (p. 233), or something else. The T wave is the most sensitive part of the tracing, and the line between normal and abnormal is not always clear.[14,222] *Low* T voltage is the most common and nonspecific of all EKG abnormalities (Fig. 13-12). Notches in T, brief interruptions of its smooth contour, may be seen in normals, especially in right precordial and transitional leads. They may represent superimposed P or merging of T and U.

Nonspecific ST-T Abnormalities

In the final analysis, all ST-T abnormalities are nonspecific. If they fit one of the patterns described above, or some other one, this is noted as a suggestion, but often they do not, and can only be

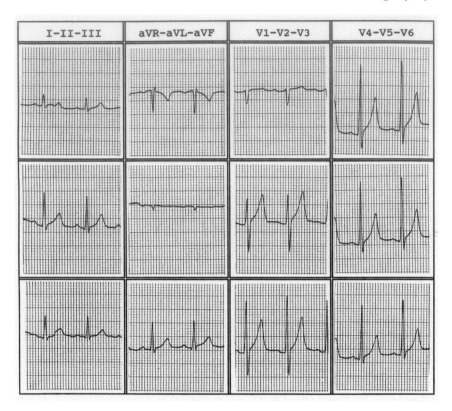

I–II–III	aVR–aVL–aVF	V1–V2–V3	V4–V5–V6

Fig. 13-11. Tall T waves.

called nonspecific. A medical student once asked what he was expected to hear when told that a tracing showed nonspecific ST-T abnormalities. A good question. The "nonspecific" part seems clear enough; it means just that—nonspecific, not typical of anything, like "I don't feel too good, Doc"—and "abnormality" requires no comment. The problem is how to relate this to the patient in terms of topography, etiology, and/or manifestations, and the answer is implicit in Dr. Wilson's observation that electrocardiographic abnormalities are not diseases (p. 5). ST-T abnormalities are statistics; their significance depends on their stability or instability, and the clinical setting in which they are observed. Dr. Lamb[19] emphasized their nonspecificity by comparing them to elevation of the sedimenta-

I-II-III	aVR-aVL-aVF	V1-V2-V3	V4-V5-V6

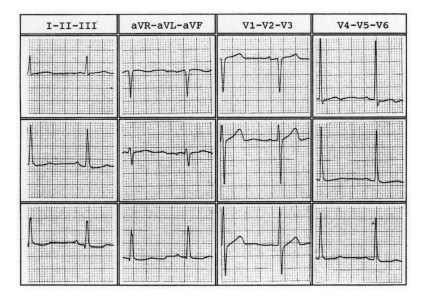

Fig. 13-12. Low T waves.

tion rate, but there is an important difference between ST-T abnormalities and the sedimentation rate. The sedimentation rate is a number reported by a technician to a doctor who interprets it as one datum among many, but nonspecific ST-T abnormalities represent evaluation by one person of information for use by another, more like nausea. Nausea is a common complaint, clearly abnormal, but subjective, a name chosen by the patient to describe a symptom in a way understood by the doctor. So what does nausea mean? It implies dysfunction of the stomach, an exceedingly complex structure that can respond to stimuli from many sources but in only a very limited number of ways, and can be evaluated only as it relates to a bigger picture. The same is true of repolarization of the ventricles. It can be modified by any of many, many factors originating in many sites, anything from ice water or hyperventilation to a myocardial infarct, from one beer too many to subarachnoid hemorrhage, and if the response is not in the form of a pattern that suggests an explanation, it is nonspecific. What this means to the patient is what the doctor has to decide on the basis of what is

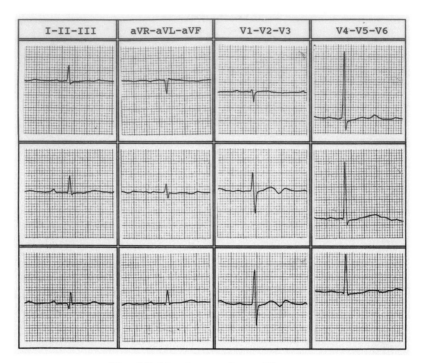

| I–II–III | aVR–aVL–aVF | V1–V2–V3 | V4–V5–V6 |

Fig. 13-13. A prominent U wave.

known from all sources, including accumulated experience with patients and electrocardiograms. Nonspecific ST-T abnormalities are found occasionally in healthy people (p. 236). To assume that they represent ischemia is inappropriate, and a potentially serious mistake. They may have no clinical implication at all.

Miscellaneous

Alternation of T amplitude from beat to beat is a rare phenomenon and of uncertain significance (p. 233).[471,545,671]

Mitral valve prolapse is often associated with negative T in leads II, III, and F, a pattern very similar to that of left ventricular overload but seen from below instead of from the left,[693] and with prolongation of QT.[776]

The U Wave

The origin of the U wave is not well understood. It has been assumed to originate in ventricular repolarization,[51,52,670] and this is probably still valid, but recently the possibility that delayed after-potentials from depolarization may be involved has been suggested (p. 184).[929] It is almost parallel to T in its spatial orientation, and duration and contour cannot be measured usefully. Abnormality is expressed as prominence, or as reversal of polarity. Negative U waves in any lead are abnormal, and, though nonspecific, correlate well with coronary insufficiency.[766,767,774] Prominence of U (Fig. 13-13) is especially common with electrolyte imbalance (p. 231) and as part of the long QT syndrome (p. 234).

FOURTEEN

Selected Topics

Tests for Reserve of Coronary Blood Supply

Studies designed to evaluate the functional reserve of a system are called *provocative*, *tolerance*, or *stress tests*. They differ from simple measurements in that they have two variables, challenge and response, both of which must be defined, one fixed, and the other validated by correlation with a criterion accepted as a measure of the reserve in question—in this case, delivery of blood, really oxygen, to the myocardium.

The diagnosis of angina pectoris is based ultimately on the history, but the underlying problem is almost always impairment of coronary blood flow by atherosclerosis, and laboratory evidence of either the anatomic lesion and/or its probable cause is helpful. Narrowing of the lumen can be demonstrated by angiographic studies, the premise that it is caused by atherosclerosis is supported by the presence of factors known to correlate with atherogenesis, as well as by evidence of the disease in other vascular beds, and radionuclide studies can show localized impairment of blood flow, but the only way yet available to show the functional lesion itself, discrepancy between supply and demand for oxygen at the cellular level, is the electrocardiogram, and the hallmark of this is transient ST displacement during pain, or in response to a controlled challenge.

The Challenge

An ideal stress test involves a single function, and a specific response to a specific stress, but in the case of biological systems this is not possible. Controlled discrepancy between supply and demand for blood in the ventricular myocardium depends on either diminishing supply or increasing demand, and, whichever method

219

is used, other functions are bound to be involved, especially respiration and the musculoskeletal system. Limitation of supply has been achieved by reduction of inspired oxygen,[314] application of ice water to an extremity,[313] and narrowing of coronary lumina by ergonovine,[602,603] but most approaches have involved increase in demand. Tachycardia induced by artificial pacing[315,316,842] has the advantage of not requiring understanding or physical action by the patient, but is complex, unpleasant, and has never been popular. Nearly all stress tests depend on exercise, and are subject to limitations other than those imposed by the coronary circulation, e.g., obesity, arthritis, debility, lung disease, and the understanding and cooperation of the patient. There are circumstances in which EKG response to unquantified exercise such as knee bends, climbing stairs, or just walking in the corridor can give useful information to a doctor who knows the patient and understands the limits of the method, but for quantitative results the challenge must be fixed. Except for those that use a bicycle ergometer, all the tests that have gained wide acceptance depend on walking, a physiologic activity requiring no training, and applicable to substantially the whole population at risk.

Criteria for the amount and type of exercise vary. The first widely used standards were those of Dr. Arthur M. Master, who began his work in exercise physiology in the 1920s and added the EKG component later. He recognized that it takes less discrepancy between supply and demand for blood to produce change in the EKG than it takes to produce pain, and that almost everyone who walks also climbs stairs. These two observations led him to devise, by trial and error over a period of years, a set of standards for exercise that would produce typical EKG patterns, but not pain, in patients with compromised coronary blood flow, and neither pain nor EKG change in normals. This consisted of a platform with two steps, each fifteen centimeters high, and a specified number of trips over these, adjusted for age, weight, and sex, to be accomplished in a specified time, the *Master two-step test*.[320,321,327] The steps have been replaced by a treadmill, permitting more precise and convenient calibration of exercise, but the principles have not changed.

Heart rate correlates well with myocardial oxygen utilization, and is used as an important criterion in the graded tests, as either an end point or a target, defining the level of stress at which the EKG response is to be evaluated, or as a measure of response to exercise quantified by other standards. The most widely used protocols are based on those described by Bruce for maximal stress, i.e., symptom limited,[566] and by Sheffield et al. for submaximal, i.e., rate limited.[630] Numerous modifications exist, and there are other protocols.

The Response

The relation between coronary atherosclerosis and angina pectoris is so well known that it is interesting to note that 160 years elapsed between Heberden's definitive description of the syndrome and convincing proof that it is due to myocardial ischemia.[564,786] The EKG picture associated with angina, flattened depression of ST (p. 206), is so well recognized now, though, that it is sometimes even equated with ischemia as if there were no other explanations. It is indeed explained by ischemia more frequently than by any other mechanism we know, and is the most critical criterion of a positive test, but occurs also in other circumstances, sometimes even in healthy young people with no reason to suspect coronary insufficiency.[738] What it apparently identifies in all cases is change in the electrophysiologic state of the deep part of the ventricular myocardium. When transient, and correlated with chest pain, or increased demand for blood in a patient with a history of chest pain, it is very strong evidence of coronary insufficiency.

Quantitative criteria for significance of EKG changes in these tests are arbitrary,[530] but any definition must fix two components, *displacement* and *contour* of ST. Displacement is defined as departure of the J point from the baseline and, because of the distribution of leads with relation to the heart, is usually recognized as depression. The contour typical of subendocardial injury is described as flattened. Depression is easy to measure, given a clear definition of baseline (p. 9), but there is no universally accepted criterion of flattening.

In 1958 Dr. Lepeschkin proposed a device for statement of both depression and flattening in a single figure, the QX:QT ratio.[325] This was accepted by Master,[318,322] and is the most nearly objective criterion available. A line is drawn connecting the beginning of two consecutive QRS complexes in a section of the trace in which the baseline is as stable as possible, and the point at which it crosses the ST segment is labeled X (Fig. 14-1). The time from onset of QRS to X is compared to the duration of QT. If there is no ST depression, QX simply measures the duration of QRS; a QX:QT ratio greater than 50% defines both depression and flattening. Other criteria include specified levels of the trace below the baseline at 0.06 or 0.08 s after J, apparently assuming a horizontal line through B as the baseline, and still others can be used,[631] but all require exceedingly accurate definition of points, and the limiting factors in all of them are human, the ability to define points, and the tendency to express estimates as if they were precise measurements; J, for instance, where displacement is defined, is more like a shoulder than a point. The QX:QT approach does not eliminate this problem, but reduces it to estimation of a single number. Increase in QRS amplitude following exercise has been proposed as another measure in this difficult area,[551] but has contributed little; too many factors contribute to QRS amplitude (p. 228). Exercise may produce ST elevation instead of depression,[327,328] or Q waves, arrhythmias, or changes limited to the T or U. All of these influence the experienced doctor in his evaluation of the patient, but flattened depression of ST remains the hallmark of a positive test, and there is general agreement that the more marked the displacement and flattening the greater the discrepancy of coronary blood flow. The need in all these studies for a control, a twelve-lead tracing made at rest, is clear.

Validity

Any laboratory study is useful only to the extent that it can be correlated with whatever it is interpreted to represent. Part of the reason for differences of opinion about the relative merits of exercise tests of coronary reserve is that different criteria are used for their validation, angina pectoris for some and coronary narrowing for others, and, though closely related, these are not the same thing.[558] Occlusion, or severe narrowing, of a major coronary artery was found in one study in about 40% of patients forty years of age or

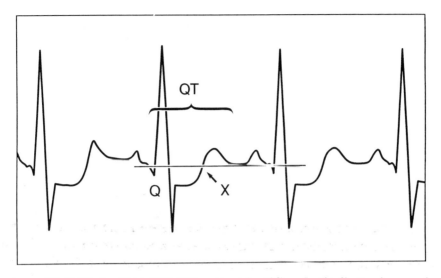

Fig. 14-1. The QX:QT ratio identifies both flattening and depression of ST (*see* p. 221).

older and free of clinical evidence of heart disease,[567] and severe narrowing may occur in healthy young adults without symptoms.[559,900] In another series, describing findings in American soldiers killed in action in their early twenties, 3% were found to have occlusive lesions of their coronary arteries.[568] The difference between the disease that is the basis for most angina, atherosclerosis, almost ubiquitous in adult Americans, and the physiologic lesion, inadequacy of oxygen supply at the cellular level, should be recognized. There may be angina without demonstrable coronary disease, and flattened ST displacement typical of subendocardial injury may be explained by means other than coronary insufficiency (p. 207).

Positive responses may occur in patients who do not have significant coronary narrowing,[784] and negative responses in those who do, no matter which test is used.[873] Digitalis,[330,537] hyperventilation,[331,500] right bundle branch block,[523,549] left bundle branch block,[499,528,565] electrolyte imbalance,[597] mitral valve prolapse,[502] and ventricular pre-excitation[332,787] may be the basis for a positive response, and in one study 20–30% of young women with no discernible heart disease had positive Master tests.[597] False positives are common in healthy young athletes.[821] The doctor who incorporates the results of an exercise test into plans for patient care must understand its limitations and use it with the same constraint that would be used with any other laboratory procedure. If a positive response is taken to mean narrowing of the lumen of a coronary artery, it is easy to define false, but, if angina pectoris is the criterion, the only way a response can be defined as false is to prove that the patient does not have angina. By the same logic, a negative response would be false if coronary narrowing were demonstrated, or if the patient really did have angina pectoris. The latter would be difficult to prove. Antianginal drugs may prevent a positive response, and so may inadequacy of the exercise stimulus.

Summary

Tests designed to evaluate the reserve of the coronary circulation vary with respect to challenge, response, and criteria for positivity. All are helpful when the question is whether chest pain is evidence of coronary insufficiency if the limitations of the method are recognized, but none is specific; all are subject to false positives and false negatives. When the cause for chest pain is in doubt, a positive stress test of any kind supports a clinical suspicion of coronary insufficiency; a negative one is against it.

The Digital Computer in Electrocardiography

By the 1950s, it was apparent that the digital computer, capable of manipulating data in tremendous volume, at great speed, and with near perfect accuracy, was well suited for analysis of electrocardiograms. Information that had been given meaning by correlation with clinical, autopsy, and experimental data accumulated over many years could be converted to numbers and analyzed rapidly and consistently. By the late 1960s, computer analysis could be had anywhere, by telephone connection to centrally located equipment, and its value was appreciated quickly. It soon became apparent, though, that, effective as it was as an aid, it did not relieve the doctor of responsibility for interpreting the tracing. It eliminates the tedium of detailed measurement, and the human error inherent in that, provides a precise and consistent base, especially helpful to one who interprets large numbers of tracings, and can make good electrocardiographers better and faster, but it can never replace judgment, never provide the final answer. A computer cannot practice medicine.[513,514,550,687,788,820]

There are two types of analysis programs, the *XYZ* or *orthogonal*, and the *twelve-lead*. The former is based on the hypothesis that all the electrical information available from any system is inherent in that projected on three mutually perpendicular leads. This is true, of course, but the usefulness of the XYZ approach is limited by the ultimately empirical nature of the subject, and the fact that all the data accumulated since the early 1900s, and validated by clinical and pathologic correlation, are based on Einthoven/Wilson methods. Twelve-lead programs are used almost exclusively, and probably will continue to be standard.

There are differences among programs just as there are differences among competitive brands of automobiles or television sets, and their relative accuracy is a matter that generates discussion. One view is that all are right all the time, if *right* is defined as doing what they have been instructed to do; the machine has no option. The relevance of the readout to the patient is another question, though, and the answer requires clinical judgment, as well as definitions; and quantitative definitions that everyone can accept, even for autopsy demonstration of such easily defined concepts as hypertrophy and infarction, are in short supply. The accuracy of a program is determined customarily by vote of a panel of experts, and some of them may be wrong,[514] or, more commonly, they don't all use exactly the same criteria. One interpreter was asked how often the computer was right when it reported "left axis deviation." His answer was "always." This was not quite what had been expected, so he added that it depends on what one means by left axis deviation *(see below)*—and the discussion came to an end. The limitation common to all programs is the human inability to digitize everything needed for interpretation, and to agree on meanings.

This problem is especially clear in disorders of impulse formation and conduction, *arrhythmias*, where distinction between description and explanation is not always respected. The amplitude and frequency of QRS are such that it can almost always be identified, even when there is a lot of background "noise," but this is not true of P waves. A computer must be told precisely how to recognize a P, how to distinguish it from a bump or wiggle, even when the trace is unstable, and, remarkable as programs are, this has not been done well enough yet to replace the human factor.[789] Contours, too, are a problem. They can be described well by adjectives understood by everyone, but are hard to reduce to numbers. Some patterns, left bundle branch block and classical myocardial infarction, for instance, can be digitized with considerable precision, but quantitative differentiation between normal and abnormal contour of ST-T is difficult.

Sometimes the information in a tracing, all by itself, can establish a diagnosis without regards to the clinical setting; second degree AV block or atrial fibrillation, for instance, but the clinical problem, and findings in previous tracings, always must be considered before a report is written. Comparison with previous tracings, and not always just the most recent one, is an absolutely necessary part of interpretation, and no programs yet available can do this effectively without human intervention.

Axis Deviation

The expression *axis deviation* has presented a problem since the beginning of electrocardiography. By long established usage, *axis* refers to projection on the frontal plane of a single value representing the net result of all energy released during ventricular depolarization. It is depicted as a ray originating at the center of the system, and is a function of both duration and amplitude of the curves, their area, not amplitude alone. *Deviation* implies that the position of this vector is outside the range of normal, left when more counterclockwise than it should be, and right when more clockwise, but no single definition of normal has been agreed upon. Those available range from complete rejection of the term[16] to "large R wave and small S wave in lead I, small R and large S wave in lead III, and frequent Q waves in lead I," a definition with no quantitative standards at all, and followed by the statement that "the validity of any other interpretation ... appears to rest upon an insecure foundation."[828]

The definition of normal as between about −30° and +105°, estimated on the basis of area determined by inspection, within limits of ±15° (p. 34), is a probably the most widely accepted one. Figures outside this range qualify as statistically abnormal but don't necessarily represent cardiac abnormality.[159,357–361] An axis counterclockwise to −30°, *left axis deviation*, may be evidence of one or more of several lesions: delay of depolarization of part of the left ventricle so that it is not counterbalanced by forces in the opposite direction that normally occur at the same time (left anterior fascicular block, p. 162), loss of muscle inferiorly (as with inferior infarction, p. 177, or hypoplasia of the left ventricle), change in electrical characteristics of the volume conductor (pulmonary emphysema, p. 232), or, probably, disproportionate increase in the mass of muscle depolarizing leftward and upward (left ventricular hypertrophy, p. 192). Structural anomalies of the chest may explain it, and so may origin of the QRS from an ectopic focus (artificial ventricular pacemaker, for instance) or poisoning, as with quinidine or potassium; it may be artifactual as a result of technical error, and sometimes it is found in the absence of any demonstrable disorder.[419] It does not correlate with obesity.[829]

Not nearly so much attention has been paid to definition of right axis deviation, probably because extremes of right axis deviation are less common than those of left. A good criterion for the clockwise limit of normal is +105°. Values greater than this are likely to be associated with right ventricular enlargement (p. 193), left posterior hemiblock (p. 165), or structural changes in the chest, but may not be abnormal at all.

Often the QRS is almost equally biphasic in all leads, frontal and precordial, and no useful figure can be given for the axis. This is called the *S1,2,3 syndrome*. It is common in normals, but may be part of the picture of right ventricular enlargement, right bundle branch block, or a myocardial infarct, and other, more complex, explanations are possible.[14,925,955]

Determinants of Voltage

Voltage is what the electrocardiogram measures, the difference in potential-to-ground between two points. There is a positive relation between the amplitude of a deflection (voltage) and the amount of energy it represents, but it is far from linear or constant; to assume, for instance, that high QRS voltage means an increase in the size of the generator, ventricular hypertrophy, and that low voltage means the opposite, is an important mistake. Myocardial mass is probably the largest single factor in determining the amplitude of a deflection,[606] but by no means the only one. The distance from myocardium to electrode is important, and the electrical properties of intervening tissues[790] influence the shape and size of the curve. Recording equipment and technique are factors, and so is the direction of the force with relation to the lead.

The volume of the ventricles influences voltage, too, some studies showing increase in voltage with increase in volume,[468,581,582] and some the opposite.[583] Myocardial ischemia has been found to diminish voltage[594] and to increase it,[591] and even myocardial infarction may increase the amplitude of the R wave,[692] but different definitions and methods are involved in these reports, and more than one interpretation can be supported in each case. Pressure itself, the product of flow and resistance, may be an important variable, voltage being greater with greater pressure,[584,585] but it may be that this should be interpreted as evidence of work instead of pressure. Voltage may be lowered by hemorrhage,[604] but then it may be restored by replacing the lost blood volume with saline. Pericardial effusion is commonly found to diminish voltage, and the mechanism for this may be diminution of the volume of blood in the ventricles, low arterial pressure, increase in venous pressure,[587,589] and/or an insulating effect of the pericardial fluid.[581,590,792–794]

Increase in the rate of flow induced by hyperthyroidism[470,593] or anemia may explain increase in voltage in some cases, and habitus has been identified as playing a role,[592] probably related to heart–electrode distance.[469] Though not very important, race and sex and age must be included in this list,[465,588] and emotional stress has been said to increase voltage.[586,593]

Criteria for high and low voltage are available in a wide range of choices. Sokolow and Lyon's definition of *high voltage*[293] (p. 193) is a convenient one. *Low voltage*[791,794] is harder to define, and generally less likely to be important; a definition that serves well is that voltage is low if the amplitude of the largest QRS, from the zenith of the tallest wave to the nadir of the deepest, in lead I, II, or III, is less than 0.5 mv. Low voltage is a statistical abnormality much as small stature is; its significance as evidence of disease depends on other factors. To say that there is low voltage in an otherwise normal electrocardiogram with a sinus mechanism at rate 50 in a patient with a hoarse voice, for instance, means something different from the same low voltage with a sinus mechanism at rate 140, blood pressure 110/100, and a paradoxical pulse. Low voltage as an incidental finding has no specific significance.

Drugs

Digitalis

Findings suggestive of digitalis effect may be seen in patients who have had none at all, and vice versa; no pattern is specific, but some are characteristic enough to be of value. The most frequent one is a certain symmetric sagging of ST combined with short QT and low T voltage; "short" is relative, but a value of less than 0.32 s at usual rates is a good reference point. The major consequences of excessive amounts of the drug are slowing of AV conduction and enhancement of ectopic activity. First degree AV block is common, and so is second degree, usually Type I (p. 152), but complete block is rare. Ectopic activity may be in the form of either PACs or PVCs, but there are many other causes for these, and, if they are manifestations of congestive failure, they may even be controlled by digitalis.[341-343] *Atrial tachycardia with block* (p. 129) may be an expression of both of these abnormalities. Other manifestations include block of conduction at the superior end of the AV node, *entrance block* (p. 146), with escape of an AV junctional pacemaker for the ventricles, and, paradoxically, acceleration of a junctional pacemaker so that it usurps pacemaker function (p. 134).

Quinidine

The effects of quinidine on the heart are complex, and some of its actions are counter to others. Typically, though, the net result is slowing of both AV and IV conduction and diminution of automaticity; it slows everything. With excess, there may be any degree of AV block, and prolongation of QRS is common (p. 168).[203,204] Theoretically, the vagolytic effect of quinidine may speed AV conduction, whereas the direct effect slows atrial rate, with the result that one-to-one conduction may occur in patients being treated for atrial flutter, so-called *1:1 flutter* (p. 131), but this is rare.

All antiarrhythmics may have, paradoxically, "proarrhythmic" effects, but, with the possible exception that these may take the form of the *torsades de pointes* pattern in ventricular fibrillation (p. 146), the electrocardiographic findings are not very helpful in identifying them as such.

Procaine amide and *disopyramide* have effects similar to quinidine.[203,600,601] *Lidocaine* produces little change.[345] *Amiodarone* may slow sinus rate and prolong PR and QRS.[795] Beta adrenergic blocking agents, *propranolol* and *nadolol*, can slow sinus rate and prolong AV and IV conduction,[344] and calcium channel blockers, *diltiazem*, *verapamil*, and *nifedipine*, have similar effects except that nifedipine does not lengthen PR. *Diphenylhydantoin* may or may not have an effect on AV conduction; the subject is controversial.[346]

Angiotensin converting enzyme (ACE) inhibitors, *captopril*, characteristically increase sinus rate.

Nitroglycerine produces no EKG changes.

Psychotropic agents can produce important findings in the electrocardiogram. The *phenothiazines* and *tricyclic antidepressants* may prolong PR, QRS, and QT, and, at toxic levels, and induce ectopy, even including ventricular fibrillation (p. 145).[348,713] It is interesting that these agents also have antiarrhythmic effects.

ST-T abnormalities seen with *chloroquine* and *emetine* may reflect abnormalities of potassium metabolism.[347] *Doxorubicin* produces cardiomyopathy in some subjects, and this may be suspected from significant reduction of the QRS voltage in serial tracings,[632] a method used also to test for evidence of rejection in cardiac transplants.

Cocaine, in therapeutic doses as a local anesthetic, produces some constriction of the coronary arteries, but no electrocardiographic changes.[951] The constriction accompanying larger doses, however, may precipitate severe impairment of blood flow and, thus, any electrocardiographic abnormality, including ventricular fibrillation, and cardiac arrest,[952] The drug also has Class I antiarrhythmic effects.

Electrolytes

Hyperkalemia produces a pattern that, when fully developed, includes tall, symmetrical, peaked T waves with diffuse widening of QRS, prolongation of PR, and, in the later stages, loss of identifiable P waves and reduction of QRS-ST-T to a smooth, continuous sine wave.[349,516] There is a rough correlation between the extent of the changes in the tracing and the concentration of potassium in the serum.[350] Hyperkalemia also may simulate left anterior hemiblock[443,516] and myocardial infarction.[249]

Hypokalemia causes lowering of T voltage, some depression of ST (in leads with positive QRS complexes), and rounding of T.[349,351] A prominent U wave may be merged with T producing a dimple in the contour of what otherwise would be called a very long QT, often seen best in right precordial leads. Whenever the QT interval is much greater than about 0.44 s, the possibility that a U wave is included in the measurement should be considered (*see Long QT syndromes*, p. 234).

The pattern of *hypocalcemia* is seen often in combination with that of hyperkalemia, and is characterized by lengthening of the QT interval with flattening of ST; changes in the sign and contour of T are inconstant.[352] With modest *hypercalcemia*, the QT is shortened, but above about 16 mg% it may be prolonged,[353] and there may be a J wave similar to the one of hypothermia (p. 237).[859] There is little change in the T wave. *Sodium, magnesium*, and other electrolytes produce little change in the electrocardiogram,[349] and changes in pH alone produce no recognizable change.[354]

The EKG patterns of electrolyte imbalance were more useful before determination of potassium and calcium levels was readily available than they are now. They still may be helpful in monitoring changes with treatment, but it is not often that the electrocardiogram will give the first clue to electrolyte imbalance.

Pulmonary Disease

Pulmonary disease can affect the electrocardiogram by several means. It can alter the electrical properties of the volume conductor, increase resistance to outflow from the right ventricle, and/or impair oxygen supply, and pain itself can produce ST-T abnormalities. These occur in a variety of patterns and may present as abnormalities of mechanism, structure, or function, either selectively or in combination.[640,641]

Disorders of mechanism are usually of atrial origin, and factors other than the lung disease may be contributory, e.g., coronary atherosclerosis, pericardial metastases. Evidence of right ventricular and/or right atrial enlargement is easy to understand as a response to increase in resistance to blood flow through the lungs, and so is precipitation of an intraventricular conduction defect.[438] The electrocardiogram is more sensitive to enlargement of the right atrium than it is to enlargement of the right ventricle, and changes in the atrium as a result of loss of compliance by the ventricle may be the first EKG evidence of overload of the right heart, visible long before there is evidence of right ventricular enlargement. Nonspecific ST-T abnormalities may be the only evidence, and there may be no abnormality at all.

Some patterns seen in pulmonary disease require comment. Prominence of Q waves in leads II, III, and AVF is particularly common, and may be a problem in the differential diagnosis of an old inferior infarct. These have been called *right atrial Q waves*,[248] but there is no really satisfactory explanation for them, and they may present a difficult problem when the complaint is chest pain. A picture suggesting an old anterior infarct may be produced, too, probably by dilatation of the right ventricle.[614] The frontal QRS may point in any direction including leftward and upward, *left axis deviation*, simulating left anterior hemiblock,[437] presumably as a result of change in intrathoracic conductance by replacement of tissue with air.[14] A classic pattern, a smooth curve from the peak of an accentuated P wave in leads II, III, and F to the peak of T, results from a combination of right atrial enlargement and ST-T abnormalities, and has been attributed to pulmonary *emphysema*.[639, 642] Pulmonary *embolism* may produce any of the patterns described above, or no EKG abnormalities at all. Findings due to it will be transient, lasting no more than hours or days.

Electrical Alternans

Electrical alternans is an unusual finding in which the amplitude of a deflection, sometimes even its sign, changes every other beat. It is seen most frequently in the QRS, but may involve any component of the tracing, selectively or in combination with others. There seems to be a temptation to attach hemodynamic significance to it, as with pulsus alternans, and it is seen sometimes with pericardial effusion, but the mechanisms responsible for it are not at all clear, and neither is its meaning. In the case of pericardial effusion, all components of the tracing are usually involved, and there may be some relation to a pendulum-like motion of the heart within the fluid, but the fundamental abnormality is probably at the cellular level. Electrical alternans is not a very important finding in the present state of our knowledge.[471,545,634–638,825,826]

Nervous System

There may be a cause-and-effect relationship between events in the nervous system and changes in the electrocardiogram.[362–365,503,595,887] EKG abnormalities resulting from CNS lesions are mostly in the ST-T complex—large, peaked T waves for instance. These may be either positive or negative in precordial leads, and may simulate those of hyperkalemia or coronary insufficiency, but peaking of T is also common in normals. Seizures, suggesting intracranial disease, may be due to third degree AV block (Stokes-Adams attacks), and muscular dystrophies may involve the heart and simulate myocardial infarction very closely (p. 182). The pattern of coronary insufficiency has been reported as reverting to normal after a cerebrovascular accident.[797] Subarachnoid hemorrhage seems especially likely to produce ST displacement, depression in most leads,[944] and meningitis may produce a similar pattern.[948] It is not clear how these effects are mediated, but autonomic influences and catecholamines must be the channels. Subendocardial hemorrhage has been reported to result from experimental chronic vagal stimulation.[945]

Blunt Trauma

Blunt trauma to the chest may produce any EKG picture, from nonspecific ST-T abnormalities through disturbances in mechanism to AV and IV conduction defects and even myocardial infarction, depending upon the location and extent of the lesion. Most of these will be transient, since they are presumably related to edema, extravasation of blood, and other intracardiac results of contusion that resolve in time.[205,252,366,369]

Congenital Heart Disease

In congenital heart disease, the electrocardiogram may help in either or both of two ways; it may point to one or more chambers as overloaded, or it may fit into a pattern, logical or not, that experience has shown to be associated with specific lesions.[372–374] Texts of cardiology are good sources of information on this subject; EKG patterns are usually included in the discussion of the various lesions and syndromes.

Long QT Syndromes

The QT interval corresponds closely with mechanical systole, and prolongation of QT, or QT-U, is very common. The clinical usefulness of this is limited because the very nature of the asymptotic ending of the curve precludes reproducibly accurate measurement, even when figures from simultaneously recorded leads are averaged over several beats (p. 201), but it is sometimes related to a propensity to ventricular fibrillation and sudden death. In 1957, Jervell and Lange-Nielsen described a constellation of findings, including a long QT interval, syncopal attacks, and congenital deafness, in four siblings, three of whom died suddenly.[695] Later, Romano et al., and Ward, noted similar findings in the absence of deafness, and other patients have been described who had QT prolongation and life-threatening arrhythmias but no identifiable hereditary basis for it. The serious problem common to all is syncope due to paroxysmal ventricular fibrillation, and the hypothesis is that the prolonged QT, or QT-U, somehow reflects the basic lesion. This may be mediated by ill-defined neurohumoral or enzymatic pathways, and current thinking links it to late after-depolarizations (p. 184). Several reviews of the syndromes have been published.[509,657,689,690,798,818,940]

Electrocardiographic Abnormalities in Healthy People

Electrocardiographic abnormalities are common in people who have no symptoms or signs of disease, and to assume that they must be evidence of structural or functional abnormality is to the patient's potential disadvantage. One of the strongest points Dr. Wilson ever made is that electrocardiographic abnormalities are not diseases, and rarely have any prognostic significance or dictate any change in lifestyle (p. 5). He emphasized this later, at a time when fear of atomic warfare was a prominent fact of life, by noting that the chance of destruction of one's "peace and happiness" by erroneous interpretation of an electrocardiogram is greater than that of being injured or killed by an atomic bomb.[935] Many studies have pointed out the frequency of electrocardiographic abnormalities in clinically healthy people *(see below)*, and the possibility that such findings will be interpreted as evidence of disease is a risk accepted by anyone who has a tracing made. Most doctors see few EKGs from patients other than their own, and, not being sensitive to the wide range of normal of each element of the tracing, many fear that every equivocal finding must be related somehow to the patient's complaints. EKG abnormalities found in healthy people include those of mechanism, P, QRS, and ST-T-U.

QRS patterns suggesting hypertrophy or dilatation of either ventricle are so common in normals that they are not likely to present much of a problem, and so are premature contractions.[707,716,870,889] Those simulating myocardial infarction have been discussed on p. 182, and other statistically defined abnormalities of orientation, duration, amplitude, and contour are encountered frequently; "incomplete right bundle branch block" and left anterior hemiblock, for instance, are common as incidental findings, and even bundle branch block may be benign (p. 171). It is especially difficult to separate first degree AV block, left atrial enlargement, left ventricular hypertrophy, and inferior myocardial infarction from normal. Too much reliance on computer readouts can be a problem.

The finding that causes perhaps more consternation than any other in healthy people is *AV block*, typically in a seventeen-year-old who presents for clearance for participation in athletics, and it can be a very perplexing problem for the clinician who has to make a decision. First degree AV block is difficult to define closely (p. 150), and third degree block can be accepted as always abnormal, but second degree block, type I (Wenckebach), is another matter when it turns up as an incidental finding in a subject with no other reason to suspect heart disease. It has been shown to occur in normal medical students going about their business,[799] and in young athletes,[824] and, in these circumstances, is thought to result from vagal and other autonomic influences, and to be benign. Long-term follow-ups of these patients are not to be found in the literature, but they are healthy people and there is no reason to think they have any greater incidence of sudden death than others.[433,734,736,739,800–803,824,830,873]

ST-T abnormalities, especially of the common garden variety, low T voltage and a little sagging of ST, are common in healthy people. They are usually unexplained and do not in themselves have prognostic significance. ST displacement, usually depression in precordial leads, is seen less commonly in normals, but does occur in the absence of any reason to suspect coronary insufficiency, especially in older people, and has been found to be transient in asymptomatic young men during Holter monitoring and exercise testing.[785,821–823,830,835,877] Elevation of ST in leads with positive QRS complexes and tall T waves is common in the absence of disease and is discussed under the heading of "early repolarization" on p. 205, and even strikingly negative precordial T waves may not be associated with any recognizable heart disease.[554,738,739,800–802,824,873]

Sleep

Very few electrocardiographic changes are found during sleep in normal people or those with coronary atherosclerosis, mostly just sinus bradycardia. In those with sleep apnea, though, a broad array of abnormalities has been identified, some of them disturbing, especially prolongation of QT, and varying degrees of AV block. No specific significance has been attached to these and presumably they relate to autonomic discharge.[804–811,836,889]

Hypothermia

Hypothermia, whether due to cold or to impairment of temperature control in the central nervous system by disease or drugs, produces a progression of EKG changes and, especially, a typical pattern that may serve as a clue to the diagnosis. This pattern is characterized by a high-frequency spike continuous with, or part of, the distal end of QRS from which it is inseparable, the *J wave of Osborn*, followed by elevation of ST and/or prolongation of QT with a negative T (Fig. 14-2). Osborn interpreted this as a "current of injury" and noted that it was almost a constant finding in dogs undergoing experimental hypothermia, preceding ventricular fibrillation by about half an hour, and related to acidosis due to "faulty elimination of CO_2." He could prevent it, as well as ventricular fibrillation, by controlling pH.[812–815] A similar wave may be seen with hypercalcemia,[859] and the similarity between this and "after-potentials" is a topic of current interest (pp. 184, 234).

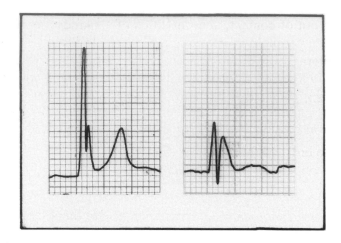

Fig. 14-2. The *J wave*, or *Osborn wave*, of hypothermia.

Pregnancy

Very little change occurs in the electrocardiogram as a result of pregnancy itself.[827,846,850]

AIDS

Cardiac involvement with the acquired immunodeficiency syndrome takes many forms,[953] but there is no typical EKG picture.

Age, Race, and Sex

The principal changes that occur with age can be described as migration of the mean QRS from clockwise and anterior in infants to counterclockwise and posterior in adults, whereas T moves in the opposite direction. The range of normal is wide, and substantially normal tracings, as judged by adult standards, may be found very early in childhood and persist to age 100 or more. Abnormalities are more frequent in the elderly, but their importance cannot be evaluated out of context; abnormalities of all kinds are more frequent in old people than in young ones.[14,465,588,737]

The literature on racial differences is small. QRS voltages may be higher in blacks than in whites, and T oriented more posteriorly, but these are generalities and not likely to be very helpful in individual cases.[824,845]

Aside from the fact that the incidence of false positive response to exercise tests is higher in women than in men,[847,848,851,852] there is no significant difference related to gender.

Appendix

The discussions of words and phrases that follow are intended to supplement the definitions beginning on p. 8, and to be helpful in describing, interpreting, and understanding electrocardiograms.

1. *Analysis*. Separation of the whole into constituent parts for individual study.

2. *Block*. Hindrance, stoppage, obstruction, or impairment of passage. For an impulse to be blocked is the opposite of its being conducted or transmitted.

   In EKG reports, block is either AV, between atria and ventricles, or IV, within a ventricle. It is evidence of discrepancy between input and output of information and may result from either diminution of the ability to conduct, demand that exceeds normal capacity for conduction, or both (*see Atrial Flutter*, p. 129).

3. *Conduct (conduction, conducted)*. To permit passage, to lead or guide from one place to another.

   The intracardiac conduction system is the network of specialized tissues over which impulses are distributed. To be conducted is the opposite of being blocked.

4. *Einthoven's premises*. The assumptions about anatomy and physiology that are the base for interpreting electrocardiograms (p. 85).

5. *Energy*. *Power* can be considered a synonym, and *force* is used almost interchangeably.

241

The concept of energy is so basic that it is hard to define, and it is probably safe to assume that everybody understands it. Energy exists in two states, potential (stored) and kinetic (active); *force* implies the latter, energy brought to bear to produce change. Whatever names are used, energy is not visible and must be represented symbolically. An electrocardiogram is a symbol of energy.

6. *Function.* Physiology, as distinguished from structure, anatomy.

7. *Galvanometer.* A device for measurement of difference in potential between two points, a voltmeter.

    A gasoline gauge in an automobile, registering the difference between zero and a value greater than zero, is an example of a galvanometer. Simplistically, an EKG machine is a galvanometer that measures the position of a point above or below a certain level, zero, and plots this against time.

8. *Ground.* A reference point, or level, an arbitrary zero for definition of potential (*see* p. 99).

    The electrical system inside the heart is not accessible to true ground, but Einthoven's premises (p. 85) define a point at the center of the chest as zero, and potentials within the body are referred to this (*see B Point*, p. 8 and *V leads*, p. 88).

9. *Interpretation.* Explanation, translation, presentation in understandable terms.

    In electrocardiography, the analytic process leading to synthesis of an evaluation; also, the product of this, the report. The report identifies mechanism, structure, and function as precisely as possible with speculation beyond that to the degree appropriate.

10. *Inverted.* Upside down, reversed in order or direction.

    T waves are often described as inverted, but this is not so accurate as indicating their direction (in degrees in the frontal plane; location of the transitional curve in the horizontal one) or indicating positivity or negativity in specified leads. Inverted does not mean negative; it implies abnormality but does not explain it.

11. *Junction.* A region of the heart, not an organ or a structure but a loosely defined area including the AV node and its vicinity.

   Impulses once thought to arise in the AV node are now said to arise in the AV junction (*see* p. 126).

12. *Lead.* Has several meanings, and, unless the intended one is selected, confusion can result.

   First, the concept of the dipole, the difference in potential between two points on the body, the unknown that the tracing documents, e.g., Lead II; second, very close to the concept but not quite the same, its graphic expression, a trace on a piece of paper; and third, a component of the patient cable, a wire, sometimes just the exploring (positive) electrode. Recognizing the difference among these is important in preventing misinterpretation of technical error as evidence of cardiac abnormality. Mislabeling of Lead II in the second sense can occur, for instance, if the piece of paper on which the trace is written is mounted in the wrong slot on a preprinted form, or upside down, even though the trace was recorded and labeled properly. Errors of mounting do not occur with multichannel recorders but leads may be mislabeled as a result of misplacement of electrodes on the body (*see* p. 104).

13. *Linear conductor.* A conductor of electricity along a linear path; an example is a wire.

   It is fundamental in electrocardiography that the arms and legs act as linear conductors attached to the volume conductor composed of the thorax and abdomen *(below)* at the shoulders and symphysis pubis.

14. *Meaning/meaningful/useful.* In the context of electrocardiography, applicable to the patient.

15. *Mechanism.* A statement of the locus of the focus driving the atria, that for the ventricles, the rate and rhythm of each, and their causal relation in a series of beats.

    Commonly called the *rhythm.*

16. *Orthogonal.* Perpendicular. *Ortho* means straight and "gonos" means angle.

    A straight angle can be defined as 180°, of course, or as 90°, and also is called a right angle—typical examples of the multiple meanings of words, in this case words on the fringes of the common language.

17. *Potential.* The possibility of force. Potential can be measured as the difference between an energy value at one level and that at another

    The potential of a volume of water, for instance, is defined in feet above sea level, that of electricity, as volts above ground—literally ground *(above).*

18. *Rhythm.* The temporal relation of events in a series, a word from everyone's everyday language.

    It has the same meaning in electrocardiography, but is used here also to refer to the several features mentioned under *Mechanism* above, features that include rhythm in the common sense of the word.

19. *Structure.* Anatomy, topography, as distinguished from function, physiology.

20. *Synthesis.* The bringing together of elements to form a whole. After a tracing has been analyzed, the parts are rearranged to synthesize an interpretation.

21. *Vector.* An arrow representing the three characteristics of force, magnitude, sense, and direction.

    The Latin word means "carrier." In strict mathematic parlance, a vector has two characteristics, magnitude and direction, is represented by a line, and is distinguished from a scalar which has only magnitude and is represented by a point. It is useful in working with electrical forces, however, and a not in conflict with this definition, to indicate a third feature, sense or polarity, origin and destination. Magnitude is represented by the length of the line, direction by its inclination, and sense by an arrowhead. An EKG is a series of values that can be thought of as the termini of a continuum of instantaneous vectors all of which arise from the same point in the center of the chest (p. 90).

22. *Volume conductor.* A system that conducts electricity in all directions at once, as distinct from a linear conductor *(above)*.

The tank full of Ringer's solution in the Physiology lab is a volume conductor. In electrocardiography, the term describes the basic premise that the thorax and abdomen comprise a volume conductor; the arms and legs, linear conductors connected to it at the shoulders and symphysis pubis. This volume conductor is assumed to be equally conductive throughout; i.e., there is no difference in the electrically conductive properties of blood, bone, liver, etc., and of infinite extent in all directions with the heart at its center *(see Einthoven's premises)*.

Bibliography

1. Wilson FN, Rosenbaum FF, Johnson FD. Interpretation of the ventricular complex of the electrocardiogram. *Adv Intern Med* 2:1, 1947.
2. Harrison TR, ed. *Principles of Internal Medicine*. Philadelphia and Toronto: Blakiston, 1950.
3. Bean WB. The natural history of error. *Arch Intern Med* 105:184, 1960.
4. Grant RP (moderator). The electrocardiogram today: A symposium discussion. *Am J Cardiol* 19:401, 1967.
5. Flowers NC, Horan LG, Tolleson WJ, et al. Localization of the site of myocardial scarring in man by high frequency components. *Circulation* 40:927, 1969.
6. Grant RP. Architectonics of the heart. *Am Heart J* 46:405, 1953.
7. Grant RP. The relationship between the anatomic position of the heart and the electrocardiogram. A criticism of "unipolar" electrocardiography. *Circulation* 7:890, 1953.
8. Mathewson FAL, Varnam GS. Abnormal electrocardiograms in apparently healthy people. I. Longterm follow-up study. *Circulation* 21:196, 1960.
9. Johnston FD. Editorial: What is a normal electrocardiogram. *Circulation* 24:707, 1961.
10. Smith HW. Plato and Clementine. *Bull NY Acad Med* 23:352, 1947.
11. Epstein FH, Doyle JT, Pollack AA, et al. Observer interpretation of electrocardiograms. *J Am Med Assoc* 175:847, 1961.
12. Caceres CA. A basis for observer variation in electrocardiographic interpretation. *Progr Cardiovasc Dis* 5:521, 1963.
13. Levine HD. Semantics and the electrocardiographic report. *Am Heart J* 65:433, 1963.
14. Beckwith JR, ed. *Grant's Clinical Electrocardiography*, 2nd ed. New York: McGraw-Hill, Blakiston Division, 1970.
15. Hurst JW, Meyerburg R. *Introduction to Electrocardiography*. New York: McGraw-Hill, Blakiston Division, 1970.
16. Katz LN. *Electrocardiography*, 2nd ed. Philadelphia: Lea and Febiger, 1946.

17. Lindsay AE, Budkin A. *The Cardiac Arrhythmias*. Chicago: Year Book Medical Publ., 1969.
18. Goldman MJ. *Principles of Clinical Electrocardiography*, 7th ed. Los Altos, California: Lange Medical Publ., 1970.
19. Lamb LE. *Electrocardiography and Vectorcardiography*. Philadelphia and London: W. B. Saunders Company, 1965.
20. Hurst JW, Logue, BR, eds. *The Heart*, 2nd ed. New York: McGraw-Hill, Blakiston Division, 1970.
21. Friedberg CK. *Diseases of the Heart*, 3rd ed. Philadelphia and London: W. B. Saunders Company, 1966.
22. Harrison TR, ed. *Principles of Internal Medicine*, 5th ed. New York: McGraw-Hill, Blakiston Division, 1966.
23. Burch GE, DePasquale NP. *A History of Electrocardiography*. Chicago: Year Book Medical Publ., 1964.
24. Waller AD. A demonstration on man of electromotive changes accompanying the heart's beat. *J Physiol* 8:229, 1887.
25. Einthoven W. Die galvanometrische Registrirung des menslichen Elektrokardiogramms zugleich eine Beurtheilung der Anwendung des Capillar-Elektrometers in der Physiologie, *Arch ges Physiol* 99:472, 1903. In Willius FA, Keys TE, eds., Translated in: *Classics of Cardiology*. New York: Henry Schuman/Dover Publ., 1961.
26. Einthoven W. Ueber die Form des menschlichen Electrocardiograms, *Arch ges Physiol* 60:101, 1895. Quoted in *Circ Res* 22:220, 1968.
27. Scherf D. Remarks on the nomenclature of cardiac arrhythmias. *Progr Cardiovasc Dis* 13:1, 1970.
28. Wolferth CC, Wood FC. The electrocardiographic diagnosis of coronary occlusion by the use of chest leads. *Am J Med Sc* 183:30, 1932.
29. Wilson FN, MacLeod AB, Barker PS. Electrocardiographic leads which record potential variations produced by the heartbeat at a single point. *Proc Soc Exp Biol Med* 29:1011, 1932.
30. Joint recommendations of the American Heart Association and the Cardiac Society of Great Britain and Ireland, a supplementary report. Standardization of precordial leads. *Am Heart J* 15:235, 1938.
31. Goldberger E. *Unipolar Lead Electrocardiography and Vectorcardiography*, 3rd ed. Philadelphia: Lea and Febiger, 1953.
32. Wilson FN, MacLeod AB, Barker PA. Electrocardiographic leads which record potential variations produced by the heartbeat at a single point. *Proc Soc Exp Biol Med* 29:1011, 1932.
33. Sherf L, James TN. A new electrocardiographic concept: Synchronized sinoventricular conduction. *Dis Chest* 55:127, 1969.

34. Emberson JW, Challice CE. Studies on the impulse conducting pathways in the atrium of the mammalian heart. *Am Heart J* 79:653, 1970.

35. James TN. The connecting pathways between the sinus node and AV node and between the right and the left atrium in the human heart. *Am Heart J* 66:498, 1963.

36. Scherf D, Cohen J. *The Atrioventricular Node and Selected Cardiac Arrhythmias.* New York: Grune and Stratton, 1964.

37. de Carvalho AP, de Mello WC, Hoffman BF, eds. *The Specialized Tissues of the Heart.* Amsterdam: Elsevier, 1961.

38. James TN. Morphology of the human atrioventricular node, with remarks pertinent to its electrophysiology. *Am Heart J* 62:756, 1961.

39. Surawicz B. Electrolytes and the electrocardiogram. *Am J Cardiol* 12:656, 1963.

40. Hoffman BF, Cranefield PF. *Electrophysiology of the Heart.* New York: Mc-Graw Hill, Blakiston Division, 1960.

41. Massumi RA, Sarin RK, Tawakkol AA, et al. Time sequence of right and left atrial depolarization as a guide to the origin of P waves. *Am J Cardiol* 24:28, 1969.

42. Hoffman BF, Moore EN, Stuckey JH, et al. Functional properties of the atrioventricular conduction system. *Circ Res* 13:308, 1963.

43. Medrano A, DeMicheli A, Cisneros F, et al. The anterior subdivision block of the left bundle branch of His. I. The ventricular activation process. *J Electrocardiol* 3:7, 1970.

44. Scher AM. The general order of ventricular excitation. In Dreifus LS, Likoff W, Moyer JH, eds., In: *Mechanisms and Therapy of Cardiac Arrhythmias.* New York and London: Grune and Stratton, 1966.

45. Fruehan CT, Baule G, Burgess MJ, et al. Differences in the heart as a generator of the QRS and ST-T deflections. *Am Heart J* 77:842, 1969.

46. Christian E, Scher AM. The effect of ventricular depolarization on the sequence of ventricular repolaration. *Am Heart J* 74:530, 1967.

47. Crain B, Burgess MJ, Millar K, et al. Observations concerning the validity of the ventricular gradient concept. *Am Heart J* 78:796, 1969.

48. Abildskov JA, Burgess MJ, Millar K, et al. New data and concepts concerning the ventricular gradient. *Chest* 58:244, 1970.

49. Simonson E, Schmitt OH, Dahl J, et al. The theoretical and experimental bases of the frontal plane ventricular gradient and its spatial counterpart. *Am Heart J* 47:122, 1954.

50. Millar K, Burgess MJ, Abildskov JA. Influence of activation order on QRST area. *Circulation* 42-III:98, 1970.

51. Lepeschkin E. The U wave of the electrocardiogram: A symposium. *Circulation* 15:68, 1957.

52. Lepeschkin E. The U wave of the electrocardiogram. *Mod Conc Cardiovasc Dis* 38:39, 1969.

53. Blake TM. The question of axis deviation. *Southern Med J* 60:1110, 1967.

54. Stinebaugh BJ, Schloeder FX, DeAlba E. An evaluation of the frontal plane QRS-T angle in normal adults. *Arch Intern Med* 116:810, 1965.

55. Burch GE, De Pasquale NP, Cronvich JA. A standard reference system for spatial vectorcardiography. Comparison of the equilateral tetrahedron and Frank systems. *Am Heart J* 80:638, 1970.

56. Burch GE, Abildskov JA, Cronvich JA. Studies of the spatial vectorcardiogram in normal man. *Circulation* 7:558, 1953.

57. Mirowski M. Ectopic rhythms originating anteriorly in the left atrium. *Am Heart J* 74:299, 1967.

58. McCaughan D, Primeau RE, Littmann D. The precordial T wave. *Am J Cardiol* 20:660, 1967.

59. Abildskov JA, Wilkinson RS Jr. The relation of precordial and orthogonal leads. *Circulation* 27:58, 1963.

60. Herbert WH, Sobol BJ. Normal atrioventricular conduction time. *Am J Med* 48:145, 1970.

61. Lepeschkin E, Surawicz B. The measurement of the duration of the QRS interval. *Am Heart J* 44:80, 1952.

62. Susmano A, Graettinger JS, Carleton RA. The relationship between QT interval and heart rate. *J Electrocardiol* 2:269, 1969.

63. Simonson E. QRS-T angle at various ages. *Circulation* 14:100, 1956.

64. Stinebaugh BJ, Schloeder FX, DeAlba E. An evaluation of the frontal plane QRS-T angle in normal adults. *Arch Intern Med* 116:810, 1965.

65. Ziegler R, Bloomfield DK. A study of the normal QRS-T angle in the frontal plane. *J Electrocardiol* 3:161, 1970.

66. Hoffman BF. Physiologic basis of disturbances of cardiac rhythm and conduction. *Progr Cardiovasc Dis* 2:319, 1959.

67. Scherf D. The mechanism of sinoatrial block. *Am J Cardiol* 23:769, 1969.

68. Greenwood RJ, Finkelstein D. *Sinoatrial Heart Block*. Springfield, IL: Charles C. Thomas, 1964.

69. Prinzmetal M, Corday E, Brill IC, et al. *The Auricular Arrhythmias*. Springfield, IL: Charles C. Thomas, 1952.

70. Scherf D. Mechanism of atrial flutter and fibrillation. In Dreifus LS, Likoff W, Moyer JH, eds., In: *Mechanisms and Therapy of Cardiac Arrhythmias*. New York: Grune and Stratton, 1966.

71. Wallace AG, Daggett WM. Re-excitation of the atrium. "The echo phenomenon." *Am Heart J* 68:661, 1964.
72. Han J. The mechanism of paroxysmal atrial tachycardia, sustained reciprocation. *Am J Cardiol* 26:329, 1970.
73. Bigger JT Jr, Goldreyer BN. The mechanism of supraventricular tachycardia. *Circulation* 42:673, 1970.
74. Choen J, Scherf D. Complete interatrial and intra-atrial block (atrial dissociation). *Am Heart J* 70:23, 1965.
75. Steffens TG. A report of atrial parasystole. *J Electrocardiol* 3:177, 1970.
76. Wit AL, Damato AN, Weill MB, et al. Phenomenon of the gap in atrioventricular conduction in the human heart. *Circ Res* 27:679, 1970.
77. Rodensky PL, Wasserman F. Atrial flutter with 1:1 conduction. *Dis Chest* 38:563, 1960.
78. Shine KI, Kastor JA, Yurchak PM. Multifocal atrial tachycardia: Clinical and electrocardiographic features. *N Engl J Med* 279:344, 1968.
79. Lipson MJ, Naimi S. Multifocal atrial tachycardia (chaotic atrial tachycardia): Clinical association and significance. *Circulation* 42:397, 1970.
80. Rosner SW. Atrial tachysystole with block. *Circulation* 29:614, 1964.
81. Lown B, Levine HD. *Atrial Arrhythmias, Digitalis, and Potassium.* New York: Landsberger Medical Books, Inc., 1952.
82. Mark H, Sham R. Nondigitalis induced paroxysmal atrial tachycardia with block. I. Management with cardioversion. *J Electrocardiol* 2:171, 1969.
83. Moore EN, Melbin J. Experimental studies on buried P waves. *J Electrocardiol* 3:1, 1970.
84. Chung EK. Atrial dissociation due to unilateral atrial fibrillation. *J Electrocardiol* 2:373, 1969.
85. Hoffman BF, Cranefield PF. The physiologic basis of cardiac arrhythmias. *Am J Med* 37:670, 1964.
86. Massumi RA. Interpolated His bundle extrasystoles. An unusual cause of tachycardia. *Am J Med* 49:265, 1970.
87. Marriott HJL, Bradley SM. Main-stem extrasystoles. *Circulation* 16:544, 1957.
88. Massumi R, Tawakkol AA. Direct study of left atrial P waves. *Am J Cardiol* 20:331, 1967.
89. Harris BC, Shaver JA, Gray S III, et al. Left atrial rhythm; experimental production in man. *Circulation* 37:1000, 1968.
90. Frankel WS, Soloff LA. Left atrial rhythm: Analysis by intraatrial electrocardiogram and the vectorcardiogram. *Am J Cardiol* 22:645, 1968.

91. Lau SH, Cohen SI, Stein E, et al. P waves and P loops in coronary sinus and left atrial ectopic rhythms. *Am Heart J* 79:201, 1970.
92. Leon DF, Lancaster JF, Shaver JA, et al. Right atrial ectopic rhythms. Experimental production in man. *Am J Cardiol* 25:6, 1970.
93. Mirowski M, Lau SH, Bobb GA, et al. Studies on left atrial automaticity in dogs. *Circ Res* 26:317, 1970.
94. Piccolo E, Nava A, Furlanello F, et al. Left atrial rhythm. Vectorcardiographic study and electrophysiologic critical evaluation. *Am Heart J* 80:11, 1970.
95. Waldo AL, Vitikainen KJ, Kaiser GA, et al. The P wave and PR interval: Effects of the site of origin of atrial depolarization. *Circulation* 42:653, 1970.
96. Damato AN, Lau SH. His bundle rhythm. *Circulation* 40:527, 1969.
97. Fisch C, Knoebel SB. Junctional rhythms. *Progr Cardiovasc Dis* 13:141, 1970.
98. Mirowski M, Tabatznik B. The spatial characteristics of atrial activation in ventriculoatrial excitation. *Chest* 57:9, 1970.
99. Marriott HLL. Retrograde doubts. *Chest* 57:2, 1970.
100. Castellanos A Jr, Castillo C, Lemberg L. His bundle electrocardiography: A programmed introduction. *Chest* 57:350, 1970.
101. Damato AN, Lau SH. Clinical value of the electrogram of the conduction system. *Progr Cardiovasc Dis* 13:119, 1970.
102. Patton RD, Stein E, Rosen KM, et al. Bundle of His electrograms: A new method for analyzing arrhythmias. *Am J Cardiol* 26:324, 1970.
103. Cohen SI, Lau SH, Berkowitz WD, et al. Concealed conduction during atrial fibrillation. *Am J Cardiol* 25:416, 1970.
104. Massumi RA, Ali N. Accelerated isorhythmic ventricular rhythms. *Am J Cardiol* 26:170, 1970.
105. Langendorff R. Concealed AV conduction: The effect of blocked impulses on the formation and conduction of subsequent impulses. *Am Heart J* 35:542, 1948.
106. Kastor JA, Yurchak PM. Recognition of digitalis intoxication in the presence of atrial fibrillation. *Ann Intern Med* 67:1045, 1967.
107. Javier RP, Narula OS, Samet P. Atrial tachysystole (flutter?) with apparent exit block. *Circulation* 40:179, 1969.
108. Pick A. Electrocardiographic features of exit-block. In Dreifus LS, Likoff W, Moyer JH, eds., In: *Mechanisms and Therapy of Cardiac Arrhythmias.* New York: Grune and Stratton, 469, 1966.
109. Damato AN, Lau SH, Bobb GA. Studies on ventriculo-atrial conduction and the re-entry phenomenon. *Circulation* 41:423, 1970.

110. Goldreyer BN, Bigger T Jr. Ventriculo-atrial conduction in man. *Circulation* 41:935, 1970.

111. Moe GK, Mendez C, Han J. Some features of a dual A-V conduction system. In Dreifus LS, Likoff W, Moyer JH, eds., In: *Mechanisms and Therapy of Cardiac Arrhythmias*. New York: Grune and Stratton, 361, 1966.

112. Wit AL, Weiss MB, Berkowitz WD, et al. Patterns of atrioventricular conduction in the human heart. *Circ Res* 27:345, 1970.

113. Roelandt J, Van der Hauwaert L. Atrial reciprocal rhythm and reciprocating tachycardia in Wolff-Parkinson-White Syndrome. *Circulation* 38:64, 1968.

114. Schamroth L, Yoshonis KF. Mechanisms in reciprocal rhythm. *Am J Cardiol* 24:224, 1969.

115. Han J. The mechanism of paroxysmal atrial tachycardia. Sustained reciprocation. *Am J Cardiol* 26:329, 1970.

116. Gulotta SJ, Aronson AL. Cardioversion of atrial tachycardia and flutter by atrial stimulation. *Am J Cardiol* 26:262, 1970.

117. Schuilenburg RM, Durrer D. Atrial echo beats in the human heart induced by atrial premature beats. *Circulation* 37:680, 1968.

118. Schuilenburg RM, Durrer D. Ventricular echo beats in the human heart elicited by induced ventricular premature beats. *Circulation* 40:337, 1969.

119. Moe GK, Childers RW, Meredith J. An appraisal of "supernormal" AV conduction. *Circulation* 38:5, 1968.

120. Mihalick M, Fisch C. Supernormal conduction of the right bundle branch. *Chest* 57:395, 1970.

121. Pick A, Langendorf R, Katz LN. The supernormal phase of atrioventricular conduction. I. Fundamental mechanisms. *Circulation* 26:388, 1962.

122. Soloff LA, Fewell JW. The supernormal phase of ventricular conduction in man. Its bearing on the genesis of ventricular premature systoles, and a note on atrioventricular conduction. *Am Heart J* 59:869, 1960.

123. Rosenbaum MB. Classification of ventricular extrasystoles according to form. *J Electrocardiol* 2:289, 1969.

124. Killip T. Dysrhythmia prophylaxis. *N Engl J Med* 281:1304, 1969.

125. Massumi RA, Tawakkol AA, Kistin AD. Re-evaluation of electrocardiographic and bedside criteria for diagnosis of ventricular tachycardia. *Circulation* 36:628, 1967.

126. Hair J, Thomas E, Eagan JT, et al. Paroxysmal ventricular tachycardia in the absence of demonstrable heart disease. *Am J Cardiol* 9:209, 1962.
127. Rosenbaum MB, Elizari MV, Lazzari JO. The mechanism of bidirectional tachycardia. *Am Heart J* 78:4, 1969.
128. Ledwich JR, Fay JE. Idiopathic recurrent ventricular fibrillation. *Am J Cardiol* 24:255, 1969.
129. Wild JB, Grover JD. The fist as an external cardiac pacemaker. *Lancet* 2:436, 1970.
130. Armbrust CA Jr, Levine SA. Paroxysmal ventricular tachycardia: A study of a hundred and seven cases. *Circulation* 1:28, 1950.
131. Herrmann GR, Park HM, Hejtmancik MR. Paroxysmal ventricular tachycardia: A clinical and electrocardiographic study. *Am Heart J* 57:166, 1959.
132. Castellanos A Jr, Lemberg L, Arcebal AG. Mechanisms of slow ventricular tachycardias in acute myocardial infarction. *Dis Chest* 56:470, 1969.
133. Deshpande SY, Magendantz HH. AV nodal parasystole associated with complete AV block. *Am J Cardiol* 23:98, 1969.
134. Scherf D, Blumenfield S, Yildoz M. Extrasystoles and parasystole. *Am Heart J* 64:357, 1962.
135. Chung EKY. Parasystole. *Progr Cardiovasc Dis* 11:64, 1968.
136. Narula OS, Samet P. Wenckebach and Mobitz type II AV block due to block within the His bundle and bundle branches. *Circulation* 41:947, 1970.
137. Rosselot E, Ahumanda J, Spoererl A, et al. Trifascicular block treated by artificial pacing. *Am J Cardiol* 26:6, 1970.
138. Harper JR, Harley A, Hackel DB, et al. Coronary artery disease and major conduction disturbances. *Am Heart J* 77:411, 1969.
139. Wenckebach KF. Zur Analyse des urregelmassingen Pulses. *Z Klin Med* 37:475, 1899.
140. Hay J. Bradycardia and cardiac arrhythmia produced by depression of certain of the functions of the heart. *Lancet* 1:139, 1906.
141. Mobitz W. Uber de unvollstandige Storung der Erregungstuberleitung zwischen Vorhof und Kammer des manschlichen Herzens. *Z Ges Exp Med* 41:180, 1924.
142. Schaffer AI. Mechanism of Wenckebach type of atrioventricular block. *Am Heart J* 79:138, 1970.
143. Langendorf R, Pick A. Atrioventricular block, Type II (Mobitz-)—its nature and clinical significance. *Circulation* 38:819, 1968.

144. Rosenbaum MB, Lepeschkin E. Bilateral bundle branch block. *Am Heart J* 50:38, 1955.
145. Schluger J, Iraj I, Edson JN. Cardiac pacing in acute myocardial infarction complicated by complete heart block. *Am Heart J* 80:116, 1970.
146. Brown RW, Hunt D, Sloman JG. The natural history of atrioventricular conduction defects in acute myocardial infarction. *Am Heart J* 78:460, 1969.
147. Feldt RH, DuShane JW, Titus JL. The atrioventricular conduction system in persistent common atrioventricular canal defect: Correlations with electrocardiogram. *Circulation* 42:437, 1970.
148. Wild JB, Grover JD. The fist as an external cardiac pacemaker. *Lancet* 2:436, 1970.
149. Rosenbaum MB. Types of right bundle branch block and their clinical significance. *J Electrocardiol* 1:221, 1968.
150. Rosenbaum MB, Elizari MV, Lazzari JO, et al. Intraventricular trifascicular blocks. The syndrome of right bundle branch block with intermittent left anterior and posterior hemiblock. *Am Heart J* 78:306, 1969.
151. Rosenbaum MB. Intraventricular trifascicular blocks. Review of the literature and classification. *Am Heart J* 78:450, 1969.
152. Sepulveda G, Rosselot E, Ahumanda J. Second degree atrioventricular block with intermittent right plus left anterior branch block. *Dis Chest* 56:553, 1969.
153. Phibbs B. Interference, dissociation, and semantics. A plea for rational nomenclature. *Am Heart J* 65:283, 1963.
154. Pick A. A-V dissociation. A proposal for a comprehensive classification and consistent terminology. *Am Heart J* 66:147, 1963.
155. Mariott HJL, Menendez MM. A-V dissociation revisited. *Progr Cardiovasc Dis* 8:522, 1966.
156. Leighton RF, Ryan JM, Goodwin RS, et al. Incomplete left bundle branch block: The view from transseptal intraventricular leads. *Circulation* 36:261, 1967.
157. Unger PN, Greenblatt M, Lev M. The anatomic basis of the electrocardiographic abnormality in incomplete left bundle branch block. *Am Heart J* 76:486, 1968.
158. Barold SS, Linhart JW, Hildner FJ, et al. Incomplete left bundle branch block: A definite electrocardiographic entity. *Circulation* 38:702, 1968.
159. Grant RP. Left axis deviation: An electrocardiographic-pathologic correlation study. *Circulation* 14:233, 1956.

160. Pryor R, Blount SG. The clinical significance of true left axis deviation. Left intraventricular blocks. *Am Heart J* 72:391, 1966.
161. Watt TB, Murao S, Pruitt RD. Left axis deviation induced experimentally in a primate heart. *Am Heart J* 70:381, 1965.
162. Rosenbaum MB. Types of left bundle branch block and their significance. *J Electrocardiol* 2:197, 1969.
163. Rosenbaum MB, Elizari MV, Levi RJ, et al. Five cases of intermittent left anterior hemiblock. *Am J Cardiol* 24:1, 1969.
164. Rosenbaum MB, Elizari MV, Lazzari JO. *The Hemiblocks*. Oldsmar, Florida: Tampa Tracings, 1970.
165. Castellanos A Jr, Maytin O, Arcebal AG, et al. Alternating and coexisting block in the divisions of the left bundle branch. *Dis Chest* 56:103, 1969.
166. Castellanos A Jr, Lemberg L, Arcebal AG, et al. Post-infarction conduction disturbances: A self-teaching program. *Dis Chest* 56:421, 1969.
167. Fernandez F, Scebat L, Lenegre J. Electrocardiographic study of left intraventricular hemiblock in man during selective coronary arteriography. *Am J Cardiol* 26:1, 1970.
168. Mariott HJL, Hogan P. Hemiblock in acute myoardial infarction. *Chest* 58:342, 1970.
169. Watt TB Jr, Pruitt R. Left posterior fascicular block in canine and primate hearts: An electrocardiographic study. *Circulation* 40:677, 1969.
170. Rosenbaum MB. Types of left bundle branch block and their clinical significance. *J Electrocardiol* 2:197, 1969.
171. Castellanos A Jr, Maytin O, Arcebal AG, et al. Significance of complete right bundle branch block with right axis deviation in absence of right ventricular hypertrophy. *Br Heart J* 32:85, 1970.
172. Dodge HT, Grant RP. Mechanisms of QRS prolongation in man. Right ventricular conduction defects. *Am J Med* 21:534, 1956.
173. Lasser RP, Haft JI, Freidberg CK. Relationship of right bundle branch block and marked left axis deviation (with left parietal or peri-infarction block) to complete heart block and syncope. *Circulation* 37:429, 1968.
174. Watt TB Jr, Pruitt RD. Character, cause, and consequence of combined left axis deviation and right bundle branch block in human electrocardiograms. *Am Heart J* 77:460, 1969.
175. Rothfield EL, Zucker IR, Tiu R, et al. The electrocardiographic syndrome of superior axis and right bundle branch block. *Dis Chest* 55:306, 1969.

176. Godman MJ, Lassers BW, Julian DG. Complete bundle branch block complicating acute myocardial infarction. *N Engl J Med* 282:237, 1970.
177. Schuilenburg RM, Durrer D. Observations on atrioventricular conduction in patients with bilateral bundle branch block. *Circulation* 41:967, 1970.
178. Narula OS, Javier RP, Samet P, et al. Significance of His and left bundle recordings from the left heart in man. *Circulation* 42:385, 1970.
179. Wolff L, Parkinson J, White PD. Bundle branch block with short PR interval in healthy young people prone to paroxysmal tachycardia. *Am Heart J* 5:685, 1930.
180. Wolff L. Wolff-Parkinson-White syndrome; historical and clinical features. *Progr Cardiovasc Dis* 2:677, 1959.
181. Ferrer I. New concepts relating to the pre-excitation syndrome. *J Am Med Assoc* 201:1038, 1967.
182. James TN. The Wolff-Parkinson-White Syndrome. *Ann Intern Med* 71:399, 1969.
183. Durrer D, Schuilenburg RM, Wellens HJJ. Pre-excitation revisited. *Am J Cardiol* 25:690, 1970.
184. James TN. The Wolff-Parkinson-White Syndrome: Evolving concepts of its pathogenesis. *Progr Cardiovasc Dis* 13:159, 1970.
185. Hejtmancik MR, Herrmann GR. The electrocardiographic syndrome of short PR interval and broad QRS complexes. *Am Heart J* 54:708, 1957.
186. Berkman NL, Lamb LE. Wolff-Parkinson-White electrocardiogram: Follow-up of five to twenty-eight years. *N Engl J Med* 278:492, 1968.
187. Castellanos A Jr, Mayer JW, Lemberg L. The electrocardiogram and vectorcardiogram in Wolff-Parkinson-White syndrome associated with bundle branch block. *Am J Cardiol* 10:657, 1962.
188. Marriott HJL, Rogers HM. Mimics of ventricular tachycardia associated with the W-P-W syndrome. *J Electrocardiol* 2:77, 1969.
189. Wasserburger RH, White DH, Lindsay ER. Noninfarctional $QS_{2,3}$ and aVF complexes as seen in the Wolff-Parkinson-White syndrome and left bundle branch block. *Am Heart J* 64:617, 1962.
190. Thomas JR. Sequential ECG changes in myocardial infarction in the W-P-W syndrome. *Dis Chest* 53:217, 1968.
191. Kulbertus HE, Collignon PG. Ventricular pre-excitation simulating anteroseptal infarction. *Dis Chest* 56:461, 1969.
192. Sodi-Pallares D, Cisneros F, Medrano GA, et al. Electrocardiographic diagnosis of myocardial infarction in the presence of bundle branch block (right and left), ventricular premature beats and Wolff-Parkinson-White syndrome. *Progr Cardiovasc Dis* 6:107, 1963.

193. Cole JS, Wills RE, Winterschied LC, et al. The Wolff-Parkinson-White syndrome: Problems in evaluation and surgical therapy. *Circulation* 42:111, 1970.

194. Cobb FR, Blumenschein SD, Sealy WC, et al. Successful surgical interruption of the bundle of Kent in a patient with Wolff-Parkinson-White syndrome. *Circulation* 38:1018, 1968.

195. Entman ML, Estes EH Jr, Hackel DB. The pathologic basis of the electrocardiographic pattern of parietal block. *Am Heart J* 74:202, 1967.

196. Corne RA, Parkin TW, Brandenburg RO, et al. Peri-infarction block: Postmyocardial-infarction intraentricular conduction disturbance. *Am Heart J* 69:150, 1965.

197. Castle CH, Keane WM. Electrocardiographic "peri-infarction block:" A clinical and pathologic correlation. *Circulation* 31:403, 1965.

198. Grant RP. Peri-infarction block. *Progr Cardiovasc Dis* 2:237, 1959.

199. Marriott HJL. Simulation of ectopic ventricular mechanisms. *J Am Med Assoc* 196:787, 1966.

200. Cohen SI, Lau SH, Haft JI, et al. Experimental production of aberrant ventricular conduction in man. *Circulation* 36:673, 1967.

201. Cohen SI, Lau SH, Stein E, et al. Variations of aberrant ventricular conduction in man: Evidence of isolated and combined block within the specialized conduction system; and electrocardiographic and vectorcardiographic study. *Circulation* 38:899, 1968.

202. Parameswaran R, Monheit R, Goldberg H. Aberrant conduction due to retrograde activation of the right bundle branch. *J Electrocardiol* 3:173, 1970.

203. Surawicz B, Lasseter KL. Effect of drugs on the electrocardiogram. *Progr Cardiovasc Dis* 13:26, 1970.

204. Heissenbuttel RH, Bigger JT Jr. The effect of oral quinidine on intraventricular conduction in man: Correlation of plasma quinidine with changes in QRS duration. *Am Heart J* 80:453, 1970.

205. Jackson DH. Transient post-traumatic right bundle branch block. *Am J Cardiol* 23:877, 1969.

206. Lewis CM, Dagenais GR, Friesinger GC, et al. Coronary aortographic appearances in patients with left bundle branch block. *Circulation* 41:299, 1970.

207. Horan LG, Flowers NC, Tolleson WJ, et al. The significance of diagnostic Q waves in the presence of bundle branch block. *Chest* 58:214, 1970.

208. Walston A II, Boineau JP, Spach MS, et al. Relationship between ventricular depolarization and QRS in right and left bundle branch block. *J Electrocardiol* 1:155, 1968.

209. Booth RW, Chou TC, Scott RC. Electrocardiographic diagnosis of ventricular hypertrophy in the presence of right bundle branch block. *Circulation* 18:169, 1958.

210. Kossman CE, Burchell HB, Pruitt RD, et al. The electrocardiogram in ventricular hypertrophy and bundle branch block. A panel discussion. *Circulation* 26:1337, 1962.

211. Scott RC. Left bundle branch block—a clinical assessment. Part III. *Am Heart J* 70:813, 1965.

212. Bauer GE. Transient bundle branch block. *Circulation* 29:730, 1964.

213. Krikler DM, Lefevre D. Intermittent left bundle branch block without obvious heart disease. *Lancet* 1:498, 1970.

214. Gooch AS, Crow RS. Labile variations of intraventricular conduction unrelated to rate changes. *Circulation* 38:480, 1968.

215. Massumi RA. Bradycardia-dependent bundle branch block: A critique and proposed criteria. *Circulation* 88:1066, 1968.

216. Sarachek NS. Bradycardia-dependent bundle branch block. Relation to supernormal conduction and phase 4 depolarization. *Am J Cardiol* 25:727, 1970.

217. Beach IB, Gracey JG, Peter RH, et al. Benign left bundle branch block. *Ann Intern Med* 70:269, 1969.

218. Bayley RH, LaDue JS. Electrocardiographic changes (local ventricular ischemia and injury), produced in the dog by temporary occlusion of a coronary artery, showing a new stage in the evolution of myocardial infarction. *Am Heart J* 27:164, 1944.

219. Bayley RH, LaDue JS. Electrocardiographic changes of impending infarction and the ischemia-injury pattern produced in the dog by total and subtotal occlusion of a coronary artery. *Am Heart J* 28:54, 1944.

220. Wasserburger RH, Corliss RJ. Prominent precordial T waves as an expression of coronary insufficiency. *Am J Cardiol* 16:195, 1965.

221. Pinto IJ, Nanda NC, Biswas AK, et al. Tall, upright T waves in the precordial leads. *Circulation* 36:708, 1967.

222. Grant RP, Estes EH Jr, Doyle JT. Spatial vector electrocardiography. The clinical characteristics of ST and T vectors. *Circulation* 3:182, 1951.

223. Caskey TD, Estes EH. Deviation of the ST segment. A review. *Am J Med* 36:424, 1964.

224. Samson WE, Scher AM. Mechanism of ST segment alteration during acute myocardial injury. *Circ Res* 8:780, 1960.

225. Bishop LH Jr, Estes EH, McIntosh HD. The electrocardiogram as a safeguard in pericardiocentesis. *J Am Med Assoc* 162:264, 1956.

226. Boineau JP, Blumenschein S, Spach MS, et al. Relationship between ventricular depolarization and electrocardiogram in myocardial infarction. *J Electrocardiol* 1:233, 1968.

227. Durrer D, Van Lier AAW, Buller J. Epicardial and intramural excitation in chronic myocardial infarction. *Am Heart J* 68:765, 1964.

228. Maxwell M, Kennamer R, Prinzmetal M. Studies on the mechanism of ventricular activity. IX. The "mural type" coronary QS wave. *Am J Med* 17:614, 1954.

229. Grant RP, Murray RH. The QRS complex deformity of myocardial infarction in the human subject. *Am J Med* 17:587, 1954.

230. Perloff JK. The recognition of strictly posterior myocardial infarction by conventional scalar electrocardiography. *Circulation* 30:706, 1964.

231. Zakopoulos KS, Tsatas AT. Old "strictly posterior" myocardial infarction. *Dis Chest* 49:545, 1966.

232. Myers GB, Klein HA, Kiratzka T. Correlation of electrocardiographic and pathologic findings in large anterolateral infarcts. *Am Heart J* 36:838, 1948.

233. Paton BC. The accuracy of diagnosis of myocardial infarction. A clinico-pathologic study. *Am J Med* 23:761, 1957.

234. Woods JD, Laurie W, Smith WG. The reliability of the electrocardiogram in myocardial infarction. *Lancet* 2:265, 1963.

235. Abbott J, Scheinman M, Schester A, et al. Correlation of clinical and EKG changes in acute myocardial infarction. *Circulation* 42(III):126, 1970.

236. Kaplan BM, Berkson DM. Serial electrocardiograms after myocardial infarction. *Ann Intern Med* 60:430, 1964.

237. Burns-Cox CJ. Return to normal of the electrocardiogram after myocardial infarction. *Lancet* 1:1194, 1967.

238. Burns-Cox CJ. The occurrence of a normal electrocardiogram after myocardial infarction. *Am Heart J* 75:572, 1968.

239. Kalbfleisch JM, Shadaksharappa KS, Conrad LL, et al. Disappearance of Q-deflection following myocardial infarction. *Am Heart J* 76:193, 1968.

240. Martinez-Rios MA, Bruto da Costa BC, Cecena-Seldner FA, et al. Normal electrocardiogram in the presence of severe coronary artery disease. *Am J Cardiol* 25:320, 1970.

241. Fulton MC, Marriott HJL. Acute pancreatitis simulating acute myocardial infarction in the electrocardiogram. *Ann Intern Med* 59:730, 1963.

242. Ruskin J, Whalen RE, Orgain ES. Electrocardiogram and vectorcardiogram simulating myocardial infarction in patient with pectus excavatum and straight back. *Am J Cardiol* 21:446, 1968.

243. Penchas S, Keynan A. Acute myocardial infarction pattern in the ECG of a patient with funnel-chest. *J Electrocardiol* 2:285, 1969.

244. Pruitt RD, Crud GW, Leachman R. Simulation of electrocardiogram of apicolateral myocardial infarction by myocardial destructive lesions of obscure etiology (myocardiopathy). *Circulation* 25:506, 1962.

245. Hamby RI, Raia F. Electrocardiographic aspects of primary myocardial disease in 60 patients. *Am Heart J* 76:316, 1968.

246. Tavel ME, Fisch C. Abnormal Q waves simulating myocardial infarction in diffuse myocardial disease. *Am Heart J* 68:534, 1964.

247. Lintermans JP, Kaplan EL, Morgan BC, et al. Infarction patterns in endocardial fibroelastosis. *Circulation* 33:202, 1966.

248. Sodi-pallares D, Biseni A, Hermann GR. Some views on the significance of qR and QR type complexes in right precordial leads in the absence of myocardial infarction. *Am Heart J* 43:716, 1952.

249. Gelzayd EA, Holzman D. Electrocardiographic changes of hyperkalemia simulating acute myocardial infarction. *Dis Chest* 51:211, 1967.

250. Klein HO, Gross H, Rubin IL. Transient electrocardiographic changes simulating myocardial infarction in open-heart surgery. *Am Heart J* 79:463, 1970.

251. Copeland RB, Omenn GS. Electrocardiogram changes suggestive of coronary artery disease in pneumothorax. *Arch Intern Med* 125:151, 1970.

252. Jones FL Jr. Transmural myocardial necrosis after nonpenetrating cardiac trauma. *Am J Cardiol* 26:419, 1970.

253. Pruitt RD, Dennis EW, Kinard S. The difficult electrocardiographic diagnosis of myocardial infarction. *Progr Cardiovasc Dis* 6:85, 1963.

254. Mamlin JJ, Weber EL, Fisch C. Electrocardiographic pattern of massive myocardial infarction without pathologic confirmation. *Circulation* 30:539, 1964.

255. Marriott HJL. Normal electrocardiographic variants simulating ischemic heart disease. *J Am Med Assoc* 199:325, 1967.

256. Beamer V, Amidi M, Scheuer J. Vectorcardiographic findings simulating myocardial infarction in aortic valve disease. *J Electrocardiol* 3:71, 1970.

257. Kini PM, Edelman EE Jr, Pipberger HV. Electrocardiographic differentiation between left ventricular hypertrophy and anterior myocardial infarction. *Circulation* 42:875, 1970.

258. Likoff W, Segal B, Dreifus L. Myocardial infarction patterns in young subjects with normal coronary arteriogram. *Circulation* 26:373, 1962.

259. Electrocardiographic infarction [editorial]. *J Am Med Assoc* 183:365, 1963.

260. Gross H, Rubin IL, Lauffer H, et al. Transient abnormal Q waves in the dog without myocardial infarction. *Am J Cardiol* 14:669, 1964.

261. Rubin IL, Gross H, Vigliano EM. Transient abnormal Q waves during coronary insufficiency. *Am Heart J* 71:254, 1966.

262. Shugoll GI. Transient QRS changes simulating myocardial infarction associated with shock and severe metabolic stress. *Am Heart J* 74:402, 1967.

263. Roesler H, Dressler W. Transient electrocardiographic changes identical with those of acute myocardial infarction accompanying attacks of angina pectoris. *Am Heart J* 47:520, 1954.

264. Phillips JH, DePasquale NP, Burch GE. The electrocardiogram in infarction of the anterolateral papillary muscle. *Am Heart J* 66:338, 1963.

265. Heikkila J. Electrocardiography in acute papillary muscle dysfunction and infarction: A clinicopathologic study. *Chest* 57:510, 1970.

266. Sano T, Ohshima H, Fujita T, et al. Correlation of ECG, VCG, and pathologic findings in subendocardial infarcts and infarct-like lesions experimentally produced by administration of substances of high molecular weight. *Am Heart J* 62:167, 1961.

267. Georas CS, Dhalquist E, Cutts FB. Subendocardial infarction: Correlation of clinical, electrocardiographic, and pathologic data in 17 cases. *Arch Intern Med* 111:488, 1963.

268. Salisbury P, Cross CE, Rieben PA. Acute ischemia of inner layers of ventricular wall. *Am Heart J* 66:650, 1963.

269. Cook RW, Edwards JE, Pruitt RD. Electrocardiographic changes in acute subendocardial infarction. I. Large subendocardial and large nontransmural infarcts. *Circulation* 18:603, 1958.

270. Cook RW, Edwards JE, Pruitt RD. Electrocardiographic changes in acute subendocardial infarction. II. Small subendocardial infarcts. *Circulation* 18:613, 1958.

271. Kostuk WJ, Beanlands DS. Complete heart block associated with acute myocardial infarction. *Am J Cardiol* 26:380, 1970.

272. Katz KH, Berk MS, Mayman CI. Acute myocardial infarction revealed in an isolated premature ventricular beat. *Circulation* 18:897, 1958.

273. Benchimol A. Myocardial infarction and ectopic beats. *J Am Med Assoc* 193:410, 1965.

274. Cohen AI. Acute myocardial infarction revealed by interpolated premature ventricular contractions. *Dis Chest* 52:83, 1967.

275. Gedge SW, Achor RWP, Berge KG, et al. Electrocardiographic and pathological study of clinically diagnosed multiple myocardial infarctions. *Circulation* 32(11):13, 1965.

276. James TN. Pathogenesis of arrhythmias in acute myocardial infarction. *Am J Cardiol* 24:791, 1969.

277. Swan HJC. Pathogenesis of arrhythmias in myocardial infarction. *Am J Cardiol* 24:836, 1969.

278. DePasquale NP. The electrocardiogram in complicated acute myocardial infarction. *Progr Cardiovasc Dis* 13:72, 1970.

279. Moyer JB, Hiller GI. Cardiac aneurysm: Clinical and electrocardiographic analysis. *Am Heart J* 41:340, 1951.

280. Flowers NC, Horan LG. Atrial infarction. *Dis Chest* 49:638, 1966.

281. Douglas AH. Atrial infarction. *Dis Chest* 54:481, 1968.

282. Dicosky C, Zimmerman HA. Atrial injury. *J Electrocardiol* 2:51, 1969.

283. Harris TR, Copeland GD, Brady DA. Progressive injury current with metastatic tumor of the heart. Case report and review of the literature. *Am Heart J* 69:392, 1965.

284. Langner PH Jr. Victims of the vector. *Am Heart J* 69:284, 1965.

285. Saha NC. Study of the P wave in normal and obstructive lung disease in Delhi. *Am Heart J* 80:154, 1970.

286. Calatayud JB, Abad JM, Khoi NB, et al. P-wave changes in chronic obstructive pulmonary disease. *Am Heart J* 79:444, 1970.

287. Morris JJ Jr, Estes EH Jr, Whalen RE, et al. P wave analysis in valvular heart disease. *Circulation* 29:242, 1964.

288. Aravalo AC, Spagnuolo M, Feinstein AR. EKG indication of left atrial enlaragement. *J Am Med Assoc* 185:358, 1963.

289. Saunders JL, Calatayud JB, Schultz KJ, et al. Evaluation of ECG criteria for P-wave abnormalities. *Am Heart J* 74:757, 1967.

290. Kasser I, Kennedy JW. The relationship of increased left atrial volume and pressure to abnormal P waves in the electrocardiogram. *Circulation* 39:339, 1969.

291. Human GP, Snyman HW. The value of the Macruz index in the diagnosis of atrial enlargement. *Circulation* 27:935, 1963.

292. Mathur VS, Levine HD. Vectorcardiographic differentiation between right ventricular hypertrophy and posterobasal myocardial infarction. *Circulation* 42:883, 1970.

293. Sokolow M, Lyon TP. The ventricular complex in left ventricular hypertrophy as obtained by unipolar precordial and limb leads. *Am Heart J* 37:161, 1949.

294. Blake TM, Dear HD. Electrocardiographic recognition of left overwork. *Southern Med J* 60:135, 1967.
295. Causey WA, Felts SK, Blake TM. Electrocardiography in the evaluation of right ventricular overload. *Southern Med J* 62:166, 1969.
296. Milnor WR. Electrocardiogram and vectorcardiogram in right ventricular hypertrophy and right bundle branch block. *Circulation* 16:348, 1957.
297. Kannel WB, Gordon T, Offutt D. Left ventricular hypertrophy by electrocardiogram. Prevalence, incidence, and mortality in the Framingham study. *Ann Intern Med* 71:89, 1969.
298. Pagnoni A, Goodwin JF. The cardiographic diagnosis of combined ventricular hypertrophy. *Br Heart J* 14:451, 1952.
299. Kossman CE, Burchell HB, Pruitt RD, et al. The electrocardiogram in ventricular hypertrophy and bundle branch block: A panel discussion. *Circulation* 26:1337, 1962.
300. Miquel C, Sodi-Pallares D, Cisneros F, et al. Right bundle branch block and right ventricular hypertrophy: Electrocardiographic and vector-cardiographic diagnosis. *Am J Cardiol* 1:57, 1958.
301. Scott RC, Norris RJ. Electrocardiographic–pathologic correlation study of left ventricular hypertrophy in the presence of left bundle branch block. *Circulation* 20:766, 1959.
302. Ostrander LD, Weinstein BJ. Electrocardiographic changes after glucose ingestion. *Circulation* 30:67, 1964.
303. Reynolds EW, Tu PN. Transmyocardial temperature gradient in dog and man: Relation to the polarity of the T wave of the electrocardiogram. *Circ Res* 15:11, 1964.
304. Kemp GL, Ellested MH. The significance of hyperventilative and orthostatic T-wave changes on the electrocardiogram. *Arch Intern Med* 121:518, 1968.
305. Mitchell JH, Shapiro AD. The relationship of adrenalin and T wave changes in anxiety state. *Am Heart J* 48:323, 1954.
306. Ostrander Jr LD. Relation of "silent" T wave inversion to cardiovascular disease in an epidemiologic study. *Am J Cardiol* 25:325, 1970.
307. Lamb LE. Electrocardiography and Vectorcardiography: Instrumentation, Fundamentals, and Clinical Application. Philadelphia and London: WB Saunders Company, 1965.
308. Blackman NS, Kuskin L. Inverted T waves in the precordial electrocardiogram of normal adolescents. *Am Heart J* 67:304, 1964.
309. Wiener L, Rios JC, Massumi RA. T wave inversion with elevated RS-T segment simulating myocardial injury. *Am Heart J* 67:684, 1964.

310. Rafailzadeh M, Luria MH, Lochaya S, et al. Physiologic studies in a healthy adolescent with inverted precordial T waves. *Dis Chest* 52:101, 1967.

311. Chou TC, Co P, Helm RA. Vectorcardiographic analysis of T wave inversion in the right precordial leads. *Am Heart J* 78:75, 1969.

312. Wasserburger RH, Alt WJ. The normal ST segment elevation variant. *Am J Cardiol* 8:184, 1961.

313. Kuaity J, Wexler H, Simonson E. The electrocardiographic ice water test. *Am Heart J* 77:569, 1969.

314. Kassebaum DG, Sutherland KI, Judkins MP. A comparison of hypoxemic and exercise electrocardiography in coronary artery disease. *Am Heart J* 75:759, 1968.

315. O'Brien KP, Higgs LM, Glancy DL, et al. Hemodynamic accompaniments of angina: A comparison during angina induced by exercise and by atrial pacing. *Circulation* 39:735, 1969.

316. Parker JO, Chiong MA, West RO, et al. Sequential alterations in myocardial lactate metabolism, ST segments, and left ventricular function during angina induced by atrial pacing. *Circulation* 40:113, 1969.

317. Simonson E. Use of the electrocardiogram in exercise tests. *Am Heart J* 66:552, 1963.

318. Master AM, Rosenfeld I. Two-step exercise test: Current status after twenty-five years. *Mod Conc Cardiovasc Dis* 36:19, 1967.

319. Master AM, Rosenfeld I. Exercise electrocardiography as an estimation of cardiac function. *Dis Chest* 51:347, 1967.

320. Master AM. The Master two-step test. *Am Heart J* 75:809, 1968.

321. Master AM, Rosenfeld I. Current status of the two-step test. *J Electrocardiol* 1:5, 1968.

322. Master AM. The Master two-step test: Some historical highlights and current concepts. *J S Carolina Med Assoc* 65(I):12, 1969.

323. Master AM. The "augmented" Master two-step test. *Circulation* 42(III):19, 1970.

324. Rosenfeld I, Master AM. Recording the electrocardiogram during the performance of the Master two-step test. *Circulation* 29:212, 1964.

325. Lepeschkin E, Surawicz B. Characteristics of true-positive and false-positive results of electrocardiographic Master two-step tests. *N Engl J Med* 258:511, 1958.

326. Robb GP, Marks HH. Latent coronary artery disease. Determination of its presence and severity by the exercise electrocardiogram. *Am J Cardiol* 13:603, 1964.

327. Master AM. ST elevation. *Am Heart J* 80:434, 1970.
328. Fortuin NJ, Friesinger GC. Exercise-induced ST segment elevation. Clinical, electrocardiographic, and arteriographic studies in twelve patients. *Am J Med* 49:459, 1970.
329. Blackburn H, Chairman. The exercise electrocardiogram. Differences in interpretation. Report of a technical group on exercise electrocardiography. *Am J Cardiol* 21:871, 1968.
330. Kawai C, Hultgran HN. The effect of digitalis upon the exercise electrocardiogram. *Am Heart J* 68:409, 1964.
331. McHenry PL, Raia F, Apiado O. False positive ECG response to exercise secondary to hyperventilation: Cineangiographic correlation. *Am Heart J* 79:683, 1970.
332. Gazes PC. False-positive exercise test in the presence of Wolff-Parkinson-White syndrome. *Am Heart J* 78:13, 1969.
333. Beard EF, Garcia E, Burke GE, et al. Postexercise electrocardiogram in screening for latent ischemic heart disease. *Dis Chest* 56:405, 1969.
334. Datey KK, Misra SN. Evaluation of two-step exercise test in patients with heart disease of different etiologies. *Dis Chest* 53:294, 1968.
335. Rowell LB, Taylor HL, Simonson E, et al. The physiologic fallacy of adjusting for body weight in performance of the Master two-step test. *Am Heart J* 70:461, 1965.
336. Sheffield LT, Reeves TJ. Graded exercise in the diagnosis of angina pectoris. *Mod Conc Cardiovasc Dis* 34:1, 1965.
337. Doan AE, Peterson DR, Blackmon JR, et al. Myocardial ischemia after maximal exercise in healthy men: One year follow-up of physically active and inactive men. *Am J Cardiol* 17:9, 1966.
338. Master AM. Is the highest rate attained in the Master "two-step" test sufficient? *Circulation* 42(III):19, 1970.
339. Goldbarg AN, Moran JF, Resnekov L. Multistage electrocardiographic exercise tests. Principles and clinical applications. *Am J Cardiol* 26:84, 1970.
340. Gutman RA, Alexander ER, Li YB, et al. Delay of ST depression after maximal exercise by walking for two minutes. *Circulation* 42:229, 1970.
341. Fisch C, Knoebel SB. Recognition and therapy of digitalis toxicity. *Progr Cardiovasc Dis* 13:71, 1970.
342. Delman AJ, Stein E. Atrial flutter secondary to digitalis toxicity. Report of three cases and review of the literature. *Circulation* 29:593, 1964.
343. Chung EK. Digitalis-induced cardiac arrhythmias. *Am Heart J* 79:845, 1970.

344. Stern S, Eisenberg S. The effect of propranolol (Inderal) on the electrocardiogram of normal subjects. *Am Heart J* 77:192, 1969.
345. Rosen KM, Lau SH, Weiss MB, et al. The effect of lidocaine on atrioventricular and intraventricular conduction in man. *Am J Cardiol* 25:1, 1970.
346. Damato AN, Berkowitz WD, Patton RD, et al. The effect of diphenyl-hydantoin on atrioventricular and intraventricular conduction in man. *Am Heart J* 79:51, 1970.
347. Sanghvi LM, Mathur BB. Electrocardiogram after chloroquine and emetine. *Circulation* 32:281, 1965.
348. Fowler NO, McCall D, Chou T-C, et al. Electrocardiographic changes and cardiac arrhythmias in patients receiving psychotropic drugs. *Am J Cardiol* 37:223, (February) 1976.
349. Surawicz B. Relationship between electrocardiogram and electrolytes. *Am Heart J* 73:814, 1967.
350. Merrill AJ. The significance of the electrocardiogram in electrolyte disturbances. *Am Heart J* 43:634, 1952.
351. Fletcher GF, Hurst JW, Schlant RC. Electrocardiographic changes in severe hypokalemia. A reappraisal. *Am J Cardiol* 20:628, 1967.
352. Bronsky D, Dubin A, Waldstein S, et al. Calcium and the electrocardiogram. I. The electrocardiographic manifestations of hypoparathyroidism. *Am J Cardiol* 7:833, 1961.
353. Bronsky D, Dubin A, Waldstein SS, et al. Calcium and the electrocardiogram. II. The electrocardiographic manifestations of hyperparathyroidism and of marked hypercalcemia from various other etiologies. *Am J Cardiol* 7:883, 1961.
354. Reid JA, Enson Y, Harvey RM, et al. The effect of variations in blood pH upon the electrocardiogram in man. *Circulation* 31:369, 1965.
355. Rohmilt D, Susilavorn B, Chou TC. Unusual electrocardiographic manifestation of pulmonary embolism. *Am Heart J* 80:237, 1970.
356. Smith M, Ray CT. Electrocardiographic signs of early right ventricular enlargement in acute pulmonary embolism. *Chest* 58:205, 1970.
357. Eliot RS, Millhon WA, Millhon J. The clinical significance of marked uncomplicated left axis deviation in men without known disease. *Am J Cardiol* 12:767, 1963.
358. Gorman PA, Calatayd JB, Abraham S, et al. Effects of age and heart disease on the QRS axis during the seventh through the tenth decades. *Am Heart J* 67:39, 1964.
359. Gup AM, Franklin RB, Hill JE Jr. The vectorcardiogram in children with left axis deviation and no apparent heart disease. *Am Heart J* 69:619, 1965.

360. Corne RA, Parkin TW, Brandenburg RO, et al. Significance of marked left axis deviation. Electrocardiographic-pathologic correlative study. *Am J Cardiol* 15:605, 1965.

361. Moller J, Carlson E, Eliot RS. Left axis deviation in children. *Dis Chest* 53:453, 1968.

362. Shirley H Jr, Davis F, Spano J. Value of the electrocardiogram in the diagnosis of intracranial disease. *Dis Chest* 53:223, 1968.

363. Falsetti HL, Willson RL. QRS voltage criteria for posterior unipolar chest leads in a normal population. *Dis Chest* 52:695, 1967.

364. Abildoskov JA, Millar K, Burgess MJ, et al. The electrocardiogram and the central nervous system. *Progr Cardiovasc Dis* 13:210, 1970.

365. Burch GE, Colcolough H, Giles T. Intracranial lesions and the heart. *Am Heart J* 80:574, 1970.

366. Dolara A, Moranda P, Pampaloni M. Electrocardiographic findings in 98 consecutive nonpenetrating chest injuries. *Dis Chest* 52:50, 1967.

367. Zinsser HF, Thind GS. Right bundle branch block after nonpenetrating injury to the chest wall. *J Am Med Assoc* 207:1913, 1969.

368. Harris LK. Transient right bundle branch block following blunt chest trauma. *Am J Cardiol* 23:884, 1969.

369. Dolara A, Pozzi L. Atrioventricular and intraventricular conduction defects after nonpenetrating trauma. *Am Heart J* 72:138, 1966.

370. Castellanos A Jr, Ortiz JM, Pastis N, et al. The electrocardiogram in patients with pacemakers. *Progr Cardiovasc Dis* 13:190, 1970.

371. Levy MN, Zieske H. Mechanism of synchronization in isorhythmic dissociation. *Circ Res* 27:429, 1970.

372. Garcia-Palmieri MR, Rodriguez RC, Girod C. The electrocardiogram and vectorcardiogram in congenital heart disease. *Am Heart J* 68:556, 1964.

373. Sodi-Pallares D (guest editor). Symposium on electrocardiography in congenital heart disease. Part I. *Am J Cardiol* 21:617, 1968.

374. Daves ML, Pryor R. Cardiac positions. *Am Heart J* 79:408, 1970.

375. Dower GE. Some instrumental errors in electrocardiography. *Circulation* 28:483, 1965.

376. Riseman JEF, Sagall EL. Diagnostic problems resulting from improper electrocardiographic technique. *J Am Med Assoc* 178:806, 1961.

377. Lepeschkin E. Electrocardiographic instrumentations. *Progr Cardiovasc Dis* 5:498, 1963.

378. Geddes LA. Where are today's pioneering manufacturers of electro-cardiographs? *J Electrocardiol* 2:1, 1969.

379. Pipberger HV. The "new" electrocardiographs: A step toward greater fidelity in recording. *Circulation* 42:771, 1970.

380. Aronow S, Bruner JMR, Siegal EF, et al. Ventricular fibrillation associated with an electrically operated bed. *N Engl J Med* 28:31, 1969.

381. Berson AS, Pipberger HV. The low-frequency response of electrocardiographs, a frequent source of recording errors. *Am Heart J* 71:779, 1966.

382. Meyer JL. Some instrument-induced errors in the electrocardiogram. *J Am Med Assoc* 201:351, 1967.

383. Berson AS, Pipberger HV. Electrocardiographic distortions caused by inadequate high-frequency response of direct writing electrocardiographs. *Am Heart J* 74:208, 1967.

384. Hirschman JC, Baker TJ, Schiff AD. Transoceanic radio transmission of electrocardiograms. *Dis Chest* 52:186, 1967.

385. Dobrow RJ, Fieldman A, Page W, et al. Transmission of electrocardiograms from a community hospital for remote computer analysis. *Am J Cardiol* 21:687, 1968.

386. Tabatznik B, Mower MM, Staewan WS. Inexpensive presentation of prolonged electrocardiographic tape recordings. *Am Heart J* 74:377, 1967.

387. Caceres CA, Hockberg HM. Performance of the computer and physician in the analysis of the electrocardiogram. *Am Heart J* 79:439, 1970.

388. Friedberg CK. Computers in cardiology. *Progr Cardiovasc Dis* 13:86, 1970.

389. Gorman PA, Evans JM. Computer analysis of the electrocardiogram: Evaluation of experience in a hospital heart station. *Am Heart J* 80:515, 1970.

390. Mattingly RF, Larks SD. The fetal electrocardiogram. *J Am Med Assoc* 183:245, 1963.

391. Buxton TM, Hsu I, Barter RH. Fetal electrocardiography. *J Am Med Assoc* 185:441, 1963.

392. Hon EH. The classification of fetal heart rate. I. A working classification. *Obstet Gynec* 22:137, 1963.

393. Ferrer MI. Instant electrocardiograms as a teaching aid. *Dis Chest* 56:344, 1969.

394. Robitaille GA, Phillips JH, Sumner RG, et al. The value of inspiratory leads in electrocardiographic diagnosis. *Dis Chest* 50:487, 1966.

395. Tranchesi J, Adelardi V, de Oliveira JM. Atrial repolarization—its importance in clinical electrocardiography. *Circulation* 22:635, 1960.

396. Starmer CF, Whalen RE, McIntosh HD. Hazards of electric shock. *Am J Cardiol* 14:537, 1964.

397. Watson H. Electrode catheters and the diagnostic application of electrocardiography in small children. *Circulation* 29:284, 1964.

398. Spach MS, Silberberg WP, Boineau JP, et al. Body surface isopotential maps in normal children, ages four to 14 years. *Am Heart J* 72:640, 1966.

399. Uhley HN. Electrocardiographic telemetry from ambulances. A practical approach to mobile coronary care units. *Am Heart J* 80:838, 1970.

400. Spangler RD, Horman MJ, Miller SW, et al. A submaximal exercise electrocardiographic test as a method of detecting occult ischemic heart disease. *Am Heart J* 80:752, 1970.

401. Smith RF, Jackson DH, Harthorne J, et al. Acquired bundle branch block in a healthy population. *Am Heart J* 80:746, 1970.

402. Awa S, Linde LM, Oshima M, et al. The significance of late-phased dart T wave in the electrocardiogram of children. *Am Heart J* 80:619, 1970.

403. Cabrera E, Gaxiola A. A critical re-evaluation of systolic and diastolic overloading patterns. *Progr Cardiovasc Dis* 2:219, 1959.

404. Kastor JA, Leinbach RC. Pacemakers and their arrhythmias. *Progr Cardiovasc Dis* 13:240, 1970.

405. Guy C, Eliot RS. The subendocardium of the left ventricle, a physiologic enigma. *Chest* 58:555, 1970.

406. Sealey WC, Boineau JP, Wallace AG. The identification and division of the bundle of Kent for premature ventricular excitation and supraventricular tachycardia. *Surgery* 68:1009, 1970.

407. Donoso E, Braunwald E, Jick S, et al. Congenital heart block. *Am J Med* 20:869, 1956.

408. Engle MA, Ehlers KH, Frand M. Natural history of congenital complete heart block, a cooperative study. *Circulation* 42(III):112, 1970.

409. Scanlon PJ, Pryor R, Blount Jr. SG. Right bundle branch block associated with left superior or inferior intraventricular block: Clinical setting, prognosis, and relation to complete heart block. *Circulation* 42:1123, 1970.

410. Scanlon PJ, Pryor R, Blount Jr. SG. Right bundle branch block associated with left superior or inferior intraventricular block: Associated with acute myocardial infarction. *Circulation* 42:1135, 1970.

411. Spach MS, Huang SN, Armstrong SI, et al. Demonstration of peripheral conduction system in human hearts. *Circulation* 38:333, 1963.

412. James TN, Sherf L. Fine structure of the His bundle. *Circulation* 44:9, 1971.
413. Cox JL, Daniel TM, Sabiston DC, et al. The electrophysiologic time-course of acute myocardial infarction and the effects of early coronary re-perfusion. *Circulation* 42(111):98, 1970.
414. Cokkinos DV, Hallman GL, Cooley DA, et al. Left ventricular aneurysm: Analysis of electrocardiographic features and postresection changes. *Am Heart J* 82:149, 1971.
415. Rochmis P, Blackburn H. Exercise tests. A survey of procedures, safety and litigation experience in approximately 170,000 tests. *J Am Med Assoc* 217:1061, 1971.
416. Okamoto N, Kaneko K, Simonson E, et al. Reliability of individual frontal plane axis determination. *Circulation* 44:213, 1971.
417. Greenspan K, Anderson GJ, Fisch C. Electrophysiologic correlates of exit block. *Am J Cardiol* 28:197, 1971.
418. Myburgh DP, Lewis BS. Ventricular parasystole in healthy hearts. *Am Heart J* 82:307, 1971.
419. Ostrander LD Jr. Left axis deviation: Prevalence, associated conditions, and prognosis. An epidemiologic study. *Ann Intern Med* 75:23, 1971.
420. Rasmussen K. Chronic sino-atrial block. *Am Heart J* 81:38, 1971.
421. Easley RM, Goldstein S. Sino-atrial syncope. *Am J Med* 50:166, 1971.
422. Gunnar RM. Cardiac conduction in patients with symptomatic sinus node disease. *Circulation* 43:836, 1971.
423. Zipes DP. Premature atrial contraction. *Arch Intern Med* 128:453, 1971.
424. Chung EK. A reappraisal of atrial dissociation. *Am J Cardiol* 28:111, 1971.
425. Damato AN, Lau SH. Concealed and supernormal AV conduction. *Circulation* 43:961, 1971.
426. Chung EK. A reappraisal of concealed atrioventricular conduction. *Am Heart J* 82:408, 1971.
427. Parker DP, Kaplan MA. Demonstration of the supernormal period in the intact human heart as a result of pacemaker failure. *Chest* 59:461, 1971.
428. Zipes DP, Fisch C. Premature ventricular beats. *Arch Intern Med* 128:140, 1971.
429. Rubenfire M, Breneman GM, Taber RE. Entrance block: A previously unrecognized phenomenon associated with transthoracic demand pacemaker implantation. *Am Heart J* 81:102, 1971.
430. Goldreyer BN, Bigger JT Jr. Site of re-entry in paroxysmal supraventricular tachycardia in man. *Circulation* 43:15, 1971.

431. Watanabe Y. Reassessment of parasystole. *Am Heart J* 81:451, 1971.
432. Proper MC, Ditchek MT, Purcell AD, et al. Nonparoxysmal bidirectional rhythm. *Chest* 59:333, 1971.
433. Perlman LV, Ostrander LD Jr, Keller JB, et al. An epidemiologic study of first degree atrioventricular block in Tecumseh, Michigan. *Chest* 59:40, 1971.
434. Haft JI, Weinstock M, DeGuia R. Electrophysiologic studies in Mobitz type II second degree heart block. *Am J Cardiol* 27:682, 1971.
435. Wartak J. *Computers in Electrocardiography*. Springfield, Illinois: Charles C. Thomas, 1970.
436. Caceres CA, Dreifus LS, eds. *Clinical Electrocardiography and Computers*. New York: Academic Press, 1970.
437. Stein PD, Bruce TA. Left axis deviation as an electrocardographic manifestation of acute pulmonary embolism. *J Electrocardiol* 4:67, 1971.
438. Johnson JC, Flowers ND, Horan JG. Unexplained atrial flutter: A frequent herald of pulmonary embolism. *Chest* 60:29, 1971.
439. Ohnell RF. Pre-excitation: A cardiac abnormality. Pathophysiological, pathoanatomical, and clinical studies of an excitatory spread phenomenon. *Acta Med Scand* (Supplement 152), 1944.
440. McHenry PL, Phillips JF, Fisch C, et al. Right precordial QRS pattern due to left anterior hemiblock. *Am Heart J* 81:498, 1971.
441. Horan LG, Flowers NC, Johnson JC. Significance of diagnostic Q wave of myocardial infarction. *Circulation* 43:428, 1971.
442. Peterson GV, Tikoff G. Left bundle branch block and left ventricular hypertrophy: Electrocardiographic-pathologic correlations. *Chest* 59:174, 1971.
443. Ewy GA, Karliner J, Bedynek Jr. JL. Electrocardiogarphic QRS axis shift as a manifestation of hyperkalemia. *J Am Med Assoc* 215:429, 1971.
444. Mariott HJL, Schwartz NL, Bix HH. Ventricular fusion beats. *Circulation* 26:880, 1962.
445. Kellerman JJ. Problems of exercise testing. *Chest* 59:124, 1971.
446. Cohn PF, Vokonas PS, Herman MV, et al. Post-exercise electrocardiogram in patients with abnormal resting electrocardiograms. *Circulation* 43:648, 1971.
447. Biberman L, Sarma RN, Surawicz B. T wave abnormalities during hyperventilation and isoproterenol infusion. *Am Heart J* 81:166, 1971.
448. Hanne-Paparo N, Wendkos MH, Burnner D. T wave abnormalities in the electrocardiograms of top-ranking athletes without demonstrable organic heart disease. *Am Heart J* 81:743, 1971.

449. Abildskov JA, Burgess MJ, Millar K, et al. The primary T wave—a new electrocardiographic wave form. *Am Heart J* 81:242, 1971.

450. Haft JI, Herman MV, Gorlin R. Left bundle branch block: Etiologic, hemodynamic, and ventriculographic considerations. *Circulation* 43:279, 1971.

451. Rosenbaum MB. The hemiblocks: Diagnostic criteria and clinical significance. *Mod Conc Cardiovasc Dis* 39:141, 1970.

452. Braudo M, Wigle ED, Keith JD. A distinctive electrocardiogram in muscular subaortic stenosis due to ventricular septal hypertrophy. *Am J Cardiol* 14:599, 1964.

453. Han J. The concepts of reentrant activity responsible for ectopic rhythms. *Am J Cardiol* 28:253, 1971.

454. Dreifus LS, Watanabe Y. Localization and significance of atrioventricular block. *Am Heart J* 82:435, 1971.

455. Piccolo E, Nava A, Della Volta S. Inferior atrial rhythms. Vectorcardiographic study and electrophysiologic considerations. *Am Heart J* 82:468, 1971.

456. Parisi AF, Beckmann CH, Lancaster MC. The spectrum of ST segment elevation in the electrocardiograms of healthy adult men. *J Electrocardiol* 4:137, 1971.

457. Zipes DP. Premature AV junctional contractions. *Arch Intern Med* 128:633, 1971.

458. Wolff L, Richman JL. The diagnosis of myocardial infarction in patients with anomalous atrioventricular excitation (Wolff-Parkinson-White syndrome). *Am Heart J* 45:545, 1953.

459. Singer DH, Eick RT. Aberrancy: Electrophysiologic aspects. *Am J Cardiol* 28:381, 1971.

460. Fisch C, Greenspan K, Anderson GJ. Exit block. *Am J Cardiol* 28:402, 1971.

461. Moore EN, Knoebel S, Spear JF. Concealed conduction. *Am J Cardiol* 28:406, 1971.

462. James TN, Sherf L. Specialized tissues and preferential conductions in the atria of the heart. *Am J Cardiol* 28:414, 1971.

463. Narula OS, Samet P. Right bundle branch block with normal, left, or right axis deviation. Analysis of His bundle recordings. *Am J Med* 51:432, 1971.

464. Zipes DP, Fisch C. Ventricular tachycardia. *Arch Intern Med* 128:815, 1971.

465. Walker ARP, Walker BF. The bearing of race, sex, age, and nutritional state on the precordial electrocardiograms of young South African Bantu and Caucasian subjects. *Am Heart J* 77:441, 1969.

466. Awa S, Linde LM, Oshima M, et al. Isolated T-wave inversion in the electrocardiogram of children. *Am Heart J* 81:166, 1971.

467. Ashcroft MT, Miller GJ, Beadnell HMSG, et al. A comparison of T-wave inversion, ST elevation, and RS amplitudes in precordial leads of Africans and Indians in Guyana. *Am Heart J* 81:467, 1971.

468. Ishikawa K, Berson AS, Pipberger HV. Electrocardiographic changes due to cardiac enlargement. *Am Heart J* 81:635, 1971.

469. Dougherty JD. The relation of QRS magnitude to the frontal QRS axis and the heart-electrode distance. *J Electrocardiol* 4:249, 1971.

470. Goel BG, Hanson CS, Han J. A-V conduction in hyper- and hypothyroid dogs. *Am Heart J* 83:504, 1972.

471. Wellens HJJ. Isolated electrical alternans of the T wave. *Chest* 62:319, 1972.

472. Bing OHL, McDowell JW, Hartman J, et al. Pacemaker placement by ECG monitoring. *N Engl J Med* 287:651, 1972.

473. Dower GE, Oxborne JA. Polarcardiographic study of hospital staff—abnormalities found in smokers. *J Electrocardiol* 5:273, 1972.

474. Schifrin BS. Fetal heart rate monitoring during labor. *J Am Med Assoc* 222:184, 1972.

475. Greenburg H, Antin S. 1:1 conduction in atrial flutter after intravenous injection of aminophylline. *J Electrocardiol* 5:391, 1972.

476. Sivertssen E, Jorganson L. Atrial dissociation. *Am Heart J* 85:103, 1973.

477. Frank E. An accurate, clinically practical system for spatial vectorcardiography. *Circulation* 13:737, 1956.

478. Luy G, Bahl OP, Massie E. Intermittent left bundle branch block. A study of the effects of left bundle branch block on the electrocardiographic patterns of myocardial infarction and ischemia. *Am Heart J* 85:332, 1973.

479. Perosio AM, Suarez LD, Llera JL. Atrial dissociation. *Am Heart J* 85:401, 1973.

480. Kastor JA. Digitalis intoxication in patients with atrial fibrillation. *Circulation* 47:888, 1973.

481. Cohen SI, Voukydis P. Disappearance of bundle branch block with slowing of normal heart rate. *Am Heart J* 85:727, 1973.

482. Gould L, Venkataraman L, Kumar M, et al. Pacemaker-induced electrocardiographic changes simulating myocardial infarction. *Chest* 63:829, 1973.

483. Lewis SM. "Lead thirteen" electrocardiograph. *J Am Med Assoc* 224:1533, 1973.

484. Schaal SF, Seidensticker J, Goodman R, et al. Familial right bundle branch block, left axis deviation, complete heart block, and early death. *Ann Intern Med* 79:63, 1973.

485. Khan AH, Haider R, Boughner DR, et al. Sinus rhythm with absent P waves in advanced rheumatic heart disease. *Am J Cardiol* 32:93, 1973.

486. Pennington KS. Advances in holography. *Scientific Am* 218:40, 1968.

487. Scherlag BJ, Lazzara R, Helfant R. Differentiation of "A-V junctional rhythms." *Circulation* 48:304, 1973.

488. Tzivoni D, Stern S. Electrocardiographic pattern during sleep in healthy subjects and in patients with ischemic heart disease. *J Electrocardiol* 6:225, 1973.

489. Shettigar UR, Hultgren J. Lead thirteen electrocardiography. *J Am Med Assoc* 226:78, 1973.

490. Fisch C, Zipes DP, McHenry PL. Rate dependent aberrancy. *Circulation* 48:714, 1973.

491. Dinari G, Aygen MM. Sinoventricular conduction. *N Engl J Med* 289:1238, 1973.

492. Legato MJ, Ferrer MI. Intermittent intraatrial block: Its diagnosis, incidence, and implications. *Chest* 65:243, 1974.

493. Walston A, Brewer DL, Kitchens CS, et al. The electrocardiographic manifestations of spontaneous left pneumothorax. *Ann Intern Med* 80:375, 1974.

494. Obel IWP, Cohen E, Millar RNS. Chronic symptomatic sinoatrial block: A review of 34 patients and their treatment. *Chest* 65:397, 1974.

495. Bruce RA. Methods of exercise testing. Step test, bicycle, treadmill, isometrics. *Am J Cardiol* 33:715, 1974.

496. Shettigar UR, Hultgren HN, Pfeifer J, et al. Diagnostic value of Q waves in inferior myocardial infarction. *Am Heart J* 88:170, 1974.

497. Bruce RA. Exercise electrocardiography: Pitfalls and solutions to interpretation. *Circulation* 50:1, 1974.

498. Friedman HS, Gomes JA, Tardio A, et al. Appearance of atrial rhythm with absent P wave in longstanding atrial fibrillation. *Chest* 66:172, 1974.

499. Cooksey JD, Parker BM, Bahl OD. The diagnostic contribution of exercise testing in left bundle branch block. *Am Heart J* 88:482, 1974.

500. Jacobs WF, Battle WE, Ronan JA. False-positive ST-T wave changes secondary to hyperventilation and exercise. A cineangiographic correlation. *Arch Intern Med* 81:479, 1974.

501. Gradboys TB, Majzoub JA. Smudge ECG. *N Engl J Med* 292:50, 1975.

502. Tuqan SK, Mau RD, Schwartz MJ. Anterior myocardial infarction patterns in the mitral valve prolapse-systolic click syndrome. *Am J Med* 58:719, 1975.

503. Hammer WJ, Luessenhop AJ, Weintraub AM. Observations on electrocardiographic changes associated with subarachnoid hemorrhage with special reference to their genesis. *Am J Med* 59:427, 1975.

504. Nizet PM, Borgia JF, Horvath SM. Wandering atrial pacemaker (prevalence in French Hornists). *J Electrocardiol* 9(1):51, 1976.

505. Stuart RH Jr, Ellestad MH. Upsloping ST segments in exercise stress testing. Six year follow-up study of 438 patients and correlation with 248 angiograms. *Am J Cardiol* 37:19, 1976.

506. Engel TR, Bond RC, Schaal SF. First degree sino-atrial heart block: Sinoatrial block in the sick-sinus syndrome. *Am Heart J* 91:303, 1976.

507. Massing GK, James TN. Anatomical configuration of the His bundle and bundle branch in the human heart. *Circulation* 53:609, 1976.

508. Das G. Left axis deviation: A spectrum of intraventricular conduction block. *Circulation* 53:917, 1976.

509. Chaudron JM, Heller F, Van den Berghe HB, et al. Attacks of ventricular fibrillation and unconsciousness in a patient with prolonged QT intrval. A family study. *Am Heart J* 91:783, 1976.

510. Kambara H, Phillip J. Long-term evaluation of early repolarization syndrome (normal variant RS-T segment elevation). *Am J Cardiol* 38:157, 1976.

511. Farnham DJ, Shah PM. Left anterior hemiblock simulating anteroseptal myocardial infarction. *Am Heart J* 92:363, 1976.

512. Spodick DH. Pericarditis vs early repolarization: Electrocardiographic differentiation. *N Engl J Med* 295:523, 1976.

513. Bertrand CA. Computer analysis of the electrocardiogram. *Am J Cardiol* 38:394, 1976.

514. Caceres CA. Limitations of computer in electrocardiographic interpretation. *Am J Cardiol* 38:362, 1976.

515. Sheffield LT, Reitman D. Stress testing methodology. *Progr Cardiovasc Dis* 19:33, 1976.

516. Arnsdorff MF. Electrocardiogram in hyperkalemia. *Arch Intern Med* 136:1161, 1976.

517. Kuritzky P, Goldfarb AL. Unusual electrocardiographic changes in spontaneous pneumothorax. *Chest* 70:535, 1976.

518. Kulbertus HE. Reevaluation of the prognosis of patients with LAD-RBBB. *Am Heart J* 92:665, 1976.

519. Zipes DP, Gaum WE, Genetos BC, et al. Atrial tachycardia without P waves masquerading as an AV junctional tachycardia. *Circulation* 55:253, 1977.

520. Wang K, Goldfarb BL, Gobel FL, et al. Multifocal atrial tachycardia. *Arch Intern Med* 137:161, 1977.

521. Jordan JL, Yamaguchi I, Mandel WJ. The sick sinus syndrome. *J Am Med Assoc* 237:682, 1977.

522. Wiberg TA, Richman HG, Gobel FL. The significance and prognosis of chronic bifascicular block. *Chest* 71:329, 1977.

523. Whinnery JE, Froelicher VF Jr, Stewart AJ, et al. The electrocardiographic response to maximal treadmill exercise of asymptomatic men with right bundle branch block. *Chest* 71:335, 1977.

524. Singer DH, Wicks J, Eick RET, et al. Atrial dissociation: Possible cellular electrophysiologic mechanisms. *Am J Med* 62:643, 1977.

525. Rotmensch HH, Meytes I, Terdiman R, et al. Incidence and significance of the low-voltage electrocardiogram in acute myocardial infarction. *Chest* 71:708, 1977.

526. Gupta PK, Lichstein E, Chadda KD. Follow-up studies in patients with right bundle branch block and left anterior hemiblock: Significance of H-V interval. *J Electrocardiol* 10(3):221, 1977.

527. Zohman LA, Kattus AA. Exercise testing in the diagnosis of coronary heart disease. *Am J Cardiol* 40:243, 1977.

528. Ibrahim MM, Tarazi RC, Dustan HP, et al. Electrocardiogram in evaluation of resistance to antihypertensive therapy. *Arch Intern Med* 137:1125, 1977.

529. Guyton RA, McClenathan JH, Newman GE, et al. Significance of subendocardial ST segment elevation caused by coronary stenosis in the dog. Epicardial ST segment depression, local ischemia, and subsequent necrosis. *Am J Cardiol* 40:373, 1977.

530. Rifkin RD, Hood WB. Bayesian analysis of electrocardiographic exercise stress testing. *N Engl J Med* 297:681, 1977.

531. Olveros RA, Seaworth J, Weiland FL, et al. Intermittent left anterior hemiblock during treadmill exercise test. *Chest* 72:492, 1977.

532. Mimbs JW, deMello V, Roberts R. The effect of respiration on normal and abnormal Q waves. An electrocardiographic and vectorcardiographic analysis. *Am Heart J* 94:579, 1977.

533. Ferrer MI. The sick sinus syndrome: Its status after ten years. *Chest* 72:554, 1977.

534. Hoffman I. Anterior conduction delay. *Am Heart J* 94:813, 1977.

535. Ogawa S, Dreifus LS, Osmick MJ. Longitudinal dissociation of Bachman's bundle as a mechanism of supraventricular tachycardia. *Am J Cardiol* 40:915, 1977.
536. James TN. The sinus node. *Am J Cardiol* 40:965, 1977.
537. Tokon MJ, Lee G, DeMaria AN, et al. Effects of digitalis on the exercise electrocardiogram in normal adult subjects. *Chest* 72:714, 1977.
538. Magram M, Lee Y-C. The pseudo-infarction pattern of left anterior hemiblock. *Chest* 72:771, 1977.
539. Nemati M, Doyle JT, McCaughan D, et al. The orthogonal electrocardiogram in normal women. Implications of sex differences in diagnostic electrocardiography. *Am Heart J* 95:12, 1978.
540. Iwamura N, Kodama I, Shimizu T, et al. Functional properties of the left septal Purkinje network in premature activation of the ventricular conduction system. *Am Heart J* 95:60, 1978.
541. Stephan E. Hereditary bundle branch system defect. Survey of a family with four affected generations. *Am Heart J* 95:89, 1978.
542. Faris JV, McHenry PL, Morris SN. Concepts and applications of treadmill exercise testing and the exercise electrocardiogram. *Am Heart J* 95:102, 1978.
543. Nakaya Y, Hiasa Y, Murayama Y, et al. Prominent anterior QRS forces as a manifestation of left septal fascicular block. *J Electrocardiol* 11(1):39, 1978.
544. Engel TR, Meister SG, Frankl WS. The "R-on-T" phenomenon. *Ann Intern Med* 88:221, 1978.
545. Navarro-Lopez F, Cinca J, Sanz G, et al. Isolated T wave alternans. *Am Heart J* 95:369, 1978.
546. Narula OS. The manifestation of bundle branch block due to lesions within the His bundle: A dilemma in electrocardiographic interpretations. *Chest* 73:312, 1978.
547. Dowell RT, McManus III RE. Pressure-induced cardiac enlargement in neonatal and adult rats: Left ventricular functional characteristics and evidence of cardiac muscle proliferation in the neonate. *Circ Res* 42:303, 1978.
548. Pastore JO, Yurchak PM, Janis KM, et al. The risk of advanced heart block in surgical patients with right bundle branch block and left axis deviation. *Circulation* 57:677, 1978.
549. Tanaka T, Friedman MJ, Okada RD, et al. Diagnostic value of exercise-induced ST segment depression in patients with right bundle branch block. *Am J Cardiol* 41:670, 1978.
550. Ariet M, Crevasse LE. Status report on computerized ECG analysis. *J Am Med Assoc* 239:1201, 1978.

551. Bonoris PE, Greenberg PS, Christinson GW, et al. Evaluation of R wave amplitude changes versus ST-segment depression in stress testing. *Circulation* 57:904, 1978.

552. Keller DH, Johnson JB. The T wave of the unipolar precordial electrocardiogram in normal adult Negro subjects. *Am Heart J* 44:494, 1952.

553. Wasserberger RH, Alt WJ, Lloyd CJ. The normal RS-T elevation variant. *Am J Cardiol* 8:184, 1961.

554. Lichtman J, O'Rourke R, Klein A, et al. Electrocardiogram of the athlete. Alterations simulating those of organic heart disease. *Arch Intern Med* 132:763, 1973.

555. Raunio H, Rissanen V, Jokinen C, et al. Significance of a terminal R wave in lead V1 of the electrocardiogram. *Am Heart J* 95:702, 1978.

556. HHO/ISC Task Force. Definition of terms related to cardiac rhythm. *Am Heart J* 95:796, 1978.

557. Scherlag BJ, Lazzara R, Helfant RH. Differentiation of "AV junctional rhythms." *Circulation* 48:304, 1973.

558. Friesinger GC, Smith RF. Correlation of electrocardiographic studies and arteriographic findings with angina pectoris. *Circulation* 46:1173, 1972.

559. McNamara JJ, Molt MA, Streple JF, et al. Coronary artery disease in combat casualties in Vietnam. *J Am Med Assoc* 216:1185, 1971.

560. Schubart AF, Marriott HJL, Gorten RJ. Isorhythmic dissociation. Atrioventricular dissociation with synchronization. *Am J Med* 24:209, 1958.

561. Herrick JB. An intimate account of my early experience with coronary thrombosis. *Am Heart J* 27:1, 1944.

562. Smith FM. The ligation of coronary arteries with electrocardiographic study. *Arch Intern Med* 22:8, 1918.

563. Mattingly TW. The postexercise electrocardiogram: Its value in the diagnosis and prognosis of coronary arterial disease. *Am J Cardiol* 9:395, 1962.

564. Feil H, Siegel ML. Electrocardiographic changes during attacks of angina pectoris. *Am J Med Sc* 175:255, 1928.

565. Orzan F, Garcia E, Mathur VS, et al. Is the treadmill test useful for evaluating coronary artery disease in patients with complete left bundle branch block? *Am J Cardiol* 42:36, 1978.

566. Doan AE, Peterson DR, Blackmon JR, et al. Myocardial ischemia after maximal exercise in healthy men. A method for detecting potential coronary heart disease? *Am Heart J* 69:11, 1965.

567. Blumgart HL. Coronary disease: Clinical-pathologic correlations and physiology. *Bull NY Acad Med* 27:693, 1951.

568. Enos WF, Holmes RH, Beyer J. Coronary artery disease among United States soldiers killed in action in Korea: Preliminary report. *J Am Med Assoc* 152:1090, 1953.
569. Chou T-C, Wenzke F. The importance of R on T phenomenon. *Am Heart J* 96:191, 1978.
570. Henson JR. Descartes and the ECG lettering system. *J Hist Med Allied Sci* 26:181, 1971.
571. Hayakawa SI. *Language in Thought and Action*, 3rd ed. New York: Harcourt Brace Jovanovich, 1972.
572. Weitzenbaum J. *Computer Power and Human Reason: From Judgment to Calculation.* San Francisco: WH Freemen and Company, 1976.
573. Mann H. A method of analyzing the electrocardiogram. *Arch Intern Med* 25:283, 1920.
574. Comroe JH Jr. *Retrospectroscope. Insights Into Medical Discovery.* Menlo Park, California: Von Gehr Press, 1977.
575. MacKenzie SJ. *Diseases of the Heart*, 4th ed. London: Oxford University Press, 1925.
576. Goodman LS, Gilman A. *The Pharmacological of Therapeutics*, Ed. II. New York: MacMillan, 1955.
577. Marriott HJL. *Practical Electrocardiography*, 6th ed. Baltimore: Williams and Wilkins, 1977.
578. Lamberti JJ, Silver H, Howell J, et al. Transmural gradients of experimental myocardial ischemia: Limited correlation of ultrastructure with epicardial ST segment. *Am Heart J* 96:496, 1978.
579. Norman TD, Coers CD. Cardiac hypertrophy after coronary ligation in rats. *Arch Pathol* 69:181, 1960.
580. Reiffel JA, Bigger JT. Pure anterior conduction delay: A variant "fascicular" defect. *J Electrocardiol* 11(4):315, 1978.
581. Nelson CV, Lange RL, Hecht HH, et al. Effect of intracardiac blood and of fluids of different conductivities on the magnitude of surface vectors. *Circulation* 14:977, 1956.
582. Nelson CV, Chatterjee M, Angelakos ET, et al. Model studies on the effect of the intracardiac blood on the electrocardiogram. *Am Heart J* 62:83, 1961.
583. Angelakos ET, Gokhan N. Influence of venous inflow volume on the QRS potential "in vivo." *Cardiologia* 42:377, 1963.
584. Dern PK, Pryor R, Walker SH, et al. Serial electrocardiographic changes in treated hypertensive patients with reference to voltage criteria, mean QRS vectors, and the QRS-T angle. *Circulation* 36:823, 1967.
585. Doyle AE. Electrocardiographic changes in hypertension treated by methonium compounds. *Am Heart J* 45:363, 1953.

586. Sigler LH. Abnormalities in the electrocardiogram induced by emotional strain. *Am J Cardiol* 8:807, 1961.
587. Spodick DH. Acute cardiac tamponade: Pathologic physiology, diagnosis, and management. *Progr Cardiovasc Dis* 10:84, 1967.
588. Blackburn H, Vasquez CL, Keys A. The aging electrocardiogram: A common aging process or latent coronary artery disease. *Am J Cardiol* 20:618, 1967.
589. Toney JC, Kilmen SN. Cardiac tamponade: Fluid and pressure effects on electrocardiographic changes. *Proc Soc Exp Biol Med* 121:642, 1966.
590. Wilson FN. The distribution of potential differences produced by the heartbeat within the body and at its surface. *Am Heart J* 5(3):599, 1930.
591. Hamlin RL, Pipers FS, Hellerstein HK, et al. Alterations in QRS during ischemia of the left ventricular free-wall in goats. *J Electrocardiol* 2(3):223, 1969.
592. Kilty SE, Lepeschkin E. Effect of body build on the QRS voltage of the electrocardiogram in normal men. Its significance in the diagnosis of left ventricular hypertrophy. *Circulation* 31:77, 1965.
593. Grubschmidt HA, Sokolow M. The reliability of high voltage of the QRS complex as a diagnostic sign of left ventricular hypertrophy in adults. *Am Heart J* 54:689, 1957.
594. Harris SA, Randall WC. Mechanisms underlying electrocardiographic changes observed in anoxia. *Am J Physiol* 142:452, 1944.
595. Greenspahn BR, Barzilai B, Denes P. Electrocardiographic changes in concussion. *Chest* 74:447, 1978.
596. Gould WL. Auricular fibrillation: Report on a study of a familial tendency, 1920-1956. *Arch Intern Med* 100:916, 1957.
597. Rosenfeld I. Personal communication, 1978.
598. Vismara LA, Vera Z, Miller RR, et al. Efficacy of disopyramide phosphate in the treatment of refractory ventricular tachycardia. *Am J Cardiol* 39:1027, 1977.
599. Woosley RL, Shand DG. Pharmacokinetics of antiarrhythmic drugs. *Am J Cardiol* 41:986, 1978.
600. Zipes DP, Troup PJ. New antiarrhythmic drugs. *Am J Cardiol* 41:1005, 1978.
601. Danilo P Jr. Cardiac effects of disopyramide. *Am Heart J* 92:532, 1976.
602. Helfant RH. Coronary arterial spasm and provocative testing in ischemic heart disease. *Am J Cardiol* 41:787, 1978.
603. Heupler PA Jr, Proudfit WL, Razavi M, et al. Ergonovine maleate provocative test for coronary arterial spasm. *Am J Cardiol* 41:631, 1978.

604. Manoach M, Gitter S, Grossman E, et al. Influence of hemorrhage on the QRS complex of the electrocardiogram. *Am Heart J* 82:55, 1971.

605. Toshima H, Koga Y, Kumura N. Correlations between electrocardiographic, vectorcardiographic, and echocardiographic findings in patients with left ventricular overload. *Am Heart J* 94:547, 1977.

606. Bennett D. Main determinant of ECG voltage measurements. *Am Heart J* 96:835, 1978.

607. Kenelly BM, Lane GK. Electrophysiological studies in four patients with atrial flutter with 1:1 atrioventricular conduction. *Am Heart J* 96:723, 1978.

608. Broome RA, Estes EH Jr, Orgain ES. The effects of digitoxin upon the twelve lead electrocardiogram. *Am J Med* 21:237, 1956.

609. Pick A. Digitalis and the electrocardiogram. *Circulation* 15:603, 1957.

610. Harrison DC, Fitzgerald JW, Winkle RA. Ambulatory ECG's to diagnose and treat cardiac arrhythmias. *N Engl J Med* 294:373, 1976.

611. Krasnow AZ, Bloomfield DK. Artifacts in portable electrocardiographic monitoring. *Am Heart J* 91:349, 1976.

612. Janse MJ, Anderson RH, van Capelle FJL, et al. A combined electrophysiological and anatomical study of the human fetal heart. *Am Heart J* 91:556, 1976.

613. Penchas S, Keynan A. False myocardial infarction pattern in the ECG of a patient with funnel-chest. *J Electrocardiol* 2:285, 1969.

614. Watanabe Y, Nishijima K, Richman H, et al. Vectorcardiographic and electrocardiographic differentiation between cor pulmonale and anterior wall myocardial infarction. *Am Heart J* 84:302, 1972.

615. Summers RS. The electrocardiogram as a diagnostic aid in pneumothorax. *Chest* 63:127, 1973.

616. Jackson DH, Murphy GW. Nonpenetrating cardiac trauma. *Mod Conc Cardiovasc Dis* 45:123, 1976.

617. Miller R, Ward C, Amsterdam E, et al. Focal mononucleosis myocarditis simulating myocardial infarction. *Chest* 63:102, 1973.

618. Ruskin JN, Akthar M, Damato AN, et al. Abnormal Q waves in Wolff-Parkinson-White Syndrome. Incidence and clinical significance. *J Am Med Assoc* 235:2727, 1976.

619. Roberts WC, McAllister HA Jr, Ferrans VJ. Sarcoidosis of the heart. A clinicopathologic study of 35 necropsy patients (Group I) and review of previously described necropsy patients (Group II). *Am J Med* 63:86, 1977.

620. Zatuchni J, Baute A. Duchenne electrocardiogram in myotonia congenita. *J Electrocardiol* 11(4):395, 1978.

621. Lemberg L. Coexisting left anterior hemiblock and inferior wall infarction. *Chest* 69:333, 1976.

622. Moleiro F, Mendoza I. Left anterior hemiblock of the 2:1 type in the presence of inferior wall myocardial infarction. *Chest* 69:418, 1976.

623. Hoffman I, Mehta J, Hilsenrath J, et al. Anterior conduction delay: A possible cause for prominent anterior QRS forces. *J Electrocardiol* 9(1):15, 1976.

624. Salem BI, Schnee M, Leatherman L, et al. Electrocardiographic pseudo-infarction pattern: Appearance with a large posterior pericardial effusion after cardiac surgery. *Am J Cardiol* 42:681, 1978.

625. Margolis JR, Kannel WB, Feinleib M, et al. Clinical features of unrecognized myocardial infarction—silent and symptomatic. Eighteen years follow-up: The Framingham study. *Am J Cardiol* 32:1, 1973.

626. Zeft HJ, Friedberg HD, King JF, et al. Reappearance of anterior QRS forces after coronary bypass surgery. An electrovectorcardiographic study. *Am J Cardiol* 36:163, 1975.

627. Conde CA, Meller J, Espinoza J, et al. Disappearance of abnormal Q waves after aortocoronary bypass surgery. *Am J Cardiol* 36:889, 1975.

628. Altieri P, Schaal SF. Inferior and anteroseptal myocardial infarction concealed by transient left anterior hemiblock. *J Electrocardiol* 6:257, 1973.

629. Dodek A, Neill WA. Corrected transposition of the great arteries masquerading as coronary artery disease. *Am J Cardiol* 30:910, 1972.

630. Sheffield LT, Holt JH, Reeves TJ. Exercise graded by heart rate in electrocardiographic testing for angina pectoris. *Circulation* 32:622, 1965.

631. Surawicz B, Saito S. Exercise testing for detection of myocardial ischemia in patients with abnormal electrocardiograms at rest. *Am J Cardiol* 41:943, 1978.

632. Minow RA, Benjamin RS, Lee ET, et al. QRS voltage change with adriamycin administration. *Cancer Treatment Reports* 62:931, 1978.

633. Rhinehart JJ, Lewis RB, Balcerzak SP. Adriamycin cardiotoxicity in man. *Ann Intern Med* 81:475, 1974.

634. Usher BW, Popp RL. Electrical alternans: Mechanism in pericardial effusion. *Am Heart J* 83:459, 1972.

635. Colvin J. Electrical alternans: Case report and comments on the literature. *Am Heart J* 55:513, 1958.

636. Spodick DH. Electrical alternans. *Am Heart J* 84:574, 1972.

637. Spodick DH. Electrical alternation of the hart. Its relation to the kinetics and physiology of the heart during cardiac tamponade. *Am J Cardiol* 10:155, 1962.

638. Littman D. Alternation of the heart. *Circulation* 27:280, 1963.
639. Wasserburger RH, Kelly JR, Rasmussen HK, et al. The electrocardiographic pentalogy of pulmonary emphysema. A correlation of roentgenographic findings and pulmonary function studies. *Circulation* 20:831, 1959.
640. Carilli AD, Denson LJ, Timmapuri N. Electrocardiographic estimation of pulmonary impairment in chronic obstruction lung disease. *Chest* 63:483, 1973.
641. Kamper D, Chou T-C, Fowler NO, et al. The reliability of electrocardiographic criteria for chronic obstructive lung disease. *Am Heart J* 80:445, 1970.
642. Littman D. The electrocardiographic findings in pulmonary emphysema. *Am J Cardiol* 5:339, 1960.
643. Cheng TO, Bashour TT. Striking electrocardiographic changes associated with pheochromocytoma. *Chest* 70:397, 1976.
644. Wang K, Segal M, Ward PCJ. Sudden disappearance of electrocardiographic pattern of anteroseptal myocardial infarction: Result of superimposed acute posterior infarction. *Chest* 70:402, 1976.
645. Burch GE. Of the PR segment depression and atrial infarction. *Am Heart J* 91:129, 1976.
646. Kleiner JP, Nelson WP, Boland MJ. The 12-lead electrocardiogram in exercise testing. A misleading baseline? *Arch Intern Med* 138:1572, 1978.
647. McAnulty JH, Rahimtoola S, Murphy ES, et al. A prospective study of sudden death in "high risk" bundle branch block. *N Engl J Med* 299:209, 1978.
648. Benditt DG, Pritchett ELC, Smith WM, et al. Characteristics of atrioventricular conduction and the spectrum of arrhythmias in Lown-Ganong-Levine syndrome. *Circulation* 57:454, 1978.
649. Joseph ME, Kastor JA. Supraventricular tachycardia in Lown-Ganong-Levine syndrome: Atrionodal versus intranodal reentry. *Am J Cardiol* 40:521, 1977.
650. Ferrer MI. Preexcitation. *Am J Med* 62:715, 1977.
651. Grayzel J, Angeles J. Sino-atrial block in man provoked by quinidine. *J Electrocardiol* 5:289, 1972.
652. Talano JV, Euler D, Randall WC, et al. Sinus node dysfunction. An overview with emphasis on autonomic and pharmacologic consideration. *Am J Med* 64:773, 1978.
653. Yabek SM, Swensson RE, Jarmakani JM. Electrocardiographic recognition of sinus node dysfunction in children and adults. *Circulation* 56:235, 1977.

654. Thery C, Gosselin B, Lekieffre J, et al. Pathology of sinoatrial node. Correlations with electrocardiographic findings in 111 patients. *Am Heart J* 93:735, 1977.

655. Kaplinsky E, Aronson R, Neufeld HN. Isorhythmic dissociation—a "physiological" arrhythmia. *J Electrocardiol* 10(2):179, 1977.

656. Moe GK, Jalife J, Mueller WJ, et al. A mathematical model of parasystole and its application to clinical arrhythmias. *Circulation* 56:968, 1977.

657. Moss AJ, Schwartz PJ. Sudden death and the idiopathic long Q-T syndrome. *Am J Med* 66:6, 1979.

658. Gay R, Brown DF. Bradycardia-dependent bundle branch block in acute myocardial infarction. *Chest* 64:114, 1973.

659. Simpson RJ Jr, Rosenthal HM, Rimmer RH Jr, et al. Alternating bundle branch block. *Chest* 74:447, 1978.

660. Dhingra RC, Amat-Y-Leon F, Windham C, et al. Significance of left axis deviation in patients with chronic left bundle branch block. *Am J Cardiol* 42:551, 1978.

661. Aiegman-Igra Y, Yahini JH, Goldbourt U, et al. Intraventricular conduction disturbances: A review of prevalence, etiology, and progression for ten years within a stable population of Israeli adult males. *Am Heart J* 96:669, 1978.

662. Lev M. The pathology of complete AV block. *Progr Cardiovasc Dis* 6:317, 1964.

663. Lenegre J. Etiology and pathology of bilateral bundle branch block in relation to complete heart block. *Progr Cardiovasc Dis* 6:409, 1964.

664. Eraker SA, Wickamasekeran R, Goldman S. Complete heart block with hyperthyroidism. *J Am Med Assoc* 239:1644, 1978.

665. Gambetta M, Childers RW. Rate-dependent right precordial Q waves: "Septal focal block." *Am J Cardiol* 32:196, 1973.

666. Danzig MD, Robertson TL, Webber LS, et al. Earlier onset of QRS in anterior precordial ECG leads: Precision of time interval measurements. *Circulation* 54:447, 1976.

667. Igarashi M, Ayabe T. Quantitative study of the supernormal phase of ventricular excitability in man. *Am J Cardiol* 36:292, 1975.

668. Hashimoto K, Corday E, Lang T-W, et al. Significance of ST segment elevations in acute myocardial ischemia. Evaluation with intracoronary electrode techniques. *Am J Cardiol* 37:493, 1976.

669. Wasserburger RH, Alt WJ, Lloyd CJ. The normal RS-T segment elevation variant. *Am J Cardiol* 8:184, 1961.

670. Watanabe Y. Purkinje repolarization as a possible cause of the U wave in the electrocardiogram. *Circulation* 51:1030, 1975.

671. Schwartz PJ, Malliani A. Electrical alternation of the T wave: Clinical and experimental evidence of its relationship with the sympathetic nervous system and with the long Q-T syndrome. *Am Heart J* 89:45, 1975.

672. Allen RD, Gettes LS, Phalan C, et al. Painless ST segment depression in patients with angina pectoris: Correlation with daily activities and cigarette smoking. *Chest* 69:467, 1976.

673. Flowers NC, Horan LG, Johnson JC. Anterior infarctional changes occurring during mid and late ventricular activation detectable by surface mapping techniques. *Circulation* 54:906, 1976.

674. Savage RM, Wagner GS, Ideker RE, et al. Correlation of postmortem anatomic findings with electrocardiographic changes in patients with myocardial infarction. *Circulation* 55:279, 1977.

675. Scheinman MM, Abbott JA. Clinical significance of transmural versus nontransmural electrocardiographic changes in patients with acute myocardial infarction. *Am J Med* 55:602, 1973.

676. Abbott JA, Scheinman MM. Nondiagnostic electrocardiogram in patients with acute myocardial infarction. Clinical and anatomic correlations. *Am J Med* 55:608, 1973.

677. Ali M, Cohen HC, Singer DH. ECG diagnosis of acute myocardial infarction in patients with pacemakers. *Arch Intern Med* 138:1534, 1978.

678. Akhtar M, Damato AN. Clinical uses of His bundle electrocardiography. Part I. *Am Heart J* 91:520, 1976.

679. Stern S, Tzivoni D. On artifacts in portable electrocardiographic monitoring. *Am Heart J* 94:131, 1977.

680. McGowan RL, Martin ND, Zaret BL, et al. Diagnostic accuracy of noninvasive myocardial imaging for coronary artery disease: An electrocardiograhpic and echocardiographic correlation. *Am J Cardiol* 40:6, 1977.

681. Rapaport A, Sepp AH, Brown WH. Carcinoma of the parathyroid gland with pulmonary metastases and cardiac death. *Am J Med* 28:443, 1960.

682. Gordon AJ, Vagueiro MC, Barold SS. Endocardial electrograms from pacemaker catheters. *Circulation* 38:82, 1968.

683. Greene HL. Clinical applications of His bundle electrocardiography. *J Am Med Assoc* 240:258, 1978.

684. Madias JE, Hood WB. Value and limitations of precordial ST segment mapping. *Arch Intern Med* 138:529, 1978.

685. Kennedy HL, Caralis DG. Ambulatory electrocardiography. A clinical perspective. *Ann Intern Med* 87:729, 1977.

686. Bonner RE, Schwetman HE. Computer diagnosis of electrocardiograms II. A computer program for EKG measurements. *Computers and Biomed Res* 1:366, 1968.

687. Pipberger HV, Cornfield J. What computer program to choose for clinical application: The need for consumer protection. *Circulation* 47:918, 1973.

688. Einthoven W. Le telecardiogramme. *Arch Internat de Physiol* 4(4):132, 1906.

689. Vincent GM, Abildskov JA, Burgess MJ. QT interval syndromes. *Progr Cardiovasc Dis* 16:523, 1974.

690. Schwartz PJ, Periti M, Malliani A. The long Q-T syndrome. *Am Heart J* 89:378, 1975.

691. Alboni P, Malacarne C, DeLorenzi E, et al. Right precordial Q waves due to superior fascicular block. Clinical and vectorcardiographic study. *J Electrocardiol* 12(1):41, 1979.

692. Ribeiro LGT, Louie EK, Hillis LD, et al. Early augmentation of R wave voltage after coronary occlusion: A useful index of myocardial injury. *J Electrocardiol* 12(1):89, 1978.

693. Devereux RB, Perloff JK, Reichnek N, et al. Mitral valve prolapse. *Circulation* 54:3, 1976.

694. Dhingra RC, Wyndham C, Amat-y-Leon F, et al. Incidence and site of AV block in patients with chronic bifascicular block. *Circulation* 59:238, 1979.

695. Jervell A, Lange-Nielsen F. Congenital deaf-mutism, functional heart disease with prolongation of the Q-T interval, and sudden death. *Am Heart J* 54:59, 1957.

696. Segers M, Lequime J, Denolin H. L'activitation ventriculaire precoce de certains couers hyperexeitables. Etude de l'onde delta de l'ectrocardiogramme. *Cardiologia* 8:113, 1944.

697. Chen C-H, Nobuyoshi M, Kawai C. ECG pattern of left ventricular hypertrophy in nonobstructive hypertrophic cardiomyopathy: The significance of the mid-precordial changes. *Am Heart J* 97:687, 1979.

698. Shapiro E. Engelmann and his laddergram. *Am J Cardiol* 39:464, 1977.

699. Athanassopoulos CB. Transient focal septal block. *Chest* 75:728, 1979.

700. Samojloff A. Reminiscences of the late Professor William Einthoven. *Am Heart J* 5:545, 1930.

701. Shapiro E. The first textbook of electrocardiography. Thomas Lewis: Clinical Electrocardiography. *J Am Coll Cardiol* 1:1160, 1983.

702. Schoolman HM. The role of the physician as advocate. *N Engl J Med* 296:103, 1977.

703. Willius FA. *Clinical Electrocardiograms: Their Interpretation and Significance.* Philadelphia: W. B. Saunders Company, 1929.
704. Lazzara R, Scherlag B. Electrophysiologic basis for arrhythmias in ischemic heart disease. *Am J Cardiol* 53:1B, 1984.
705. Bigger JT Jr. Antiarrhythmic treatment: An overview. *Am J Cardiol* 53:8B, 1984.
706. Guntheroth WG, Selzer A, Spodick DH. Atrioventricular nodal rhythm reconsidered. *Am J Cardiol* 52:416, 1989.
707. Horan MJ, Kennedy HL. Ventricular ectopy. History, epidemiology, and clinical importance. *J Am Med Assoc* 251:380, 1984.
708. Hiraoka M, Adaniya H. Function of atrial preferential conduction routes under normal and abnormal conditions. *J Electrocardiol* 16(2):123, 1983.
709. Woolliscroft J, Tuna N. Permanent atrial standstill: The clinical spectrum. *Am J Cardiol* 49:2037, 1982.
710. Ruff P, Leier CV, Schaal SF. Temporary atrial standstill. *Am Heart J* 98:413, 1979.
711. Santinelli V, Chiariello M, Condorelli M. Exit block during "common" atrial flutter: Convincing proof for focal origin of the arrhythmia. *Chest* 85:144, 1984.
712. Kay GN, Plumb VJ, Arciniegas JG, et al. Torsades de pointes: The long-short initiating sequence and other clinical features: Observations in 32 patients. *J Am Coll Cardiol* 2:806, 1983.
713. Marshall JB, Forker AD. Cardiovascular effects of tricyclic antidepressant drugs: Therapeutic usage, overdose, and management of complications. *Am Heart J* 103:401, (March) 1982.
714. Ludomirsky A, Klein HO, Sarelli P, et al. Q-T prolongation and polymorphous ("torsade de pointes") ventricular arrhythmias associated with organophosphorus insecticide poisoning. *Am J Cardiol* 49:1654, 1982.
715. Warner RA, Hill NE, Mookherjee S, et al. Electrocardiographic criteria for the diagnosis of combined inferior myocardial infarction and left anterior hemiblock. *Am J Cardiol* 51:723, 1983.
716. Kennedy HL, Underhill SJ. Frequent or complex ventricular ectopy in apparently healthy subjects: A clinical study of 25 cases. *Am J Cardiol* 38:141, 1976.
717. Bauman JL, Bauernfeind RA, Hoff JV, et al. Torsades de pointes due to quinidine: Observations of 31 patients. *Am Heart J* 107:425, 1984.
718. Thomas MG, Giles TD. Mexiletine: Long-term follow-up of a patient with prolonged QT interval and quinidine-induced torsades de pointes. *Southern Med J* 78:205, 1985.

719. Bar FW, Brugada P, Dassen WR, et al. Prognostic value of Q waves, R/S ratio, loss of R voltage, ST-T segment abnormalities, electrical axis, low voltage, and notching: Correlation of electrocardiogram and left ventriculogram. *J Am Coll Cardiol* 4:17, 1984.

720. Klein HO, Tordjman T, Ninio R, et al. Early recognition of right ventricular infarction: Diagnostic accuracy of the electrocardiographic V4R lead. *Circulation* 67:558, 1983.

721. Myers GB. QRS-T pattern in multiple precordial leads that may be mistaken for myocardial infarction. I. Left ventricular hypertrophy and dilatation. *Circulation* 1:844, 1950.

722. Myers GB. QRS-T pattern in multiple precordial leads that may be mistaken for myocardial infarction. II. Right ventricular hypertrophy and dilatation. *Circulation* 1:860, 1950.

723. Geft IL, Shah PK, Rodriguez L, et al. ST elevations in leads V1 to V5 may be caused by right coronary artery occlusion and acute right ventricular infarction. *Am J Cardiol* 53:991, 1984.

724. Spodick DH. Q wave infarction versus S-T infarction. *Am J Cardiol* 51:913, 1983.

725. Pipberger HV, Lopez EA. "Silent" subendocardial infarcts: Fact or fiction? *Am Heart J* 100:597, 1980.

726. Zarling EJ, Sexton H, Milnor P. Failure to diagnose acute myocardial infarction. The clinicopathologic experience at a large community hospital. *J Am Med Assoc* 250:1177, 1983.

727. Cosio FG, Moro C, Alonso M, et al. The Q waves of hypertrophic cardiomyopathy: An electrophysiologic study. *N Engl J Med* 302:96, 1980.

728. Pipberger H, Schwartz L, Massumi RA, et al. Studies on the mechanism of ventricular activity. XXI: The origin of the depolarization complex with clinical applications. *Am Heart J* 54:511, 1957.

729. Raunio H, Rissanen V, Romppanen T, et al. Changes in the QRS complex and ST segment in transmural and subendocardial myocardial infarctions. A clinicopathologic study. *Am Heart J* 98:176, 1979.

730. Phibbs B. "Transmural" versus "subendocardial" myocardial infarction: An electrocardiographic myth. *J Am Coll Cardiol* 1:561, 1983.

731. Braat SH, Brugada P, den Dulk K, et al. Value of lead V4R for recognition of the infarct coronary artery in acute inferior myocardial infarction. *Am J Cardiol* 53:1538, 1984.

732. Huang SK, Rosenberg MJ, Denes P. Short PR interval and narrow QRS complex associated with pheochromocytoma: Electrophysiologic observations. *J Am Coll Cardiol* 3:872, 1984.

733. Greene HL, Ryan RF, McKusick VA. Profound first-degree atrioventricular block. A 30-year study. *Chest* 74:212, 1978.

734. Erikssen J, Otterstad JE. Natural course of a prolonged PR interval and the relation between PR and incidence of coronary heart disease. A 7-year follow-up study of 1832 apparently healthy men aged 40–59 years. *Clin Cardiol* 7:6, 1984.

735. Strasberg B, Ashley WW, Wyndham CRC, et al. Treadmill exercise testing in the Wolff-Parkinson-White syndrome. *Am J Cardiol* 45:742, 1980.

736. Strasberg B, Amat-y-Leon F, Dhingra RC, et al. Natural history of chronic second degree atrioventricular block. *Circulation* 63:1043, 1981.

737. Mihalick MJ, Fisch C. Electrocardiographic findings in the aged. *Am Heart J* 87:117, 1974.

738. Mathewson FAL, Varnam GS. Abnormal electrocardiograms in apparently healthy people: I. Long term follow-up study. *Circulation* 21:196, 1960.

739. Mathewson FAL, Varnam GS. Abnormal electrocardiograms in apparently healthy people: II. The electrocardiogram in the diagnosis of subclinical myocardial disease. Serial records of 32 people. *Circulation* 21:204, 1960.

740. Savard P, Cohen D, Lepeschkin E, et al. Magnetic measurement of ST-T and T-Q segment shifts in humans. Part I: Early repolarization and left bundle branch block. *Circ Res* 53:264, 1983.

741. Karp PJ, Katila TE, Saarinen M, et al. The normal human magnetocardiogram: II. A multipole analysis. *Circ Res* 47:117, 1980.

742. Abildskov JA, Green LS, Lux RL. The present status of body surface mapping. *J Am Coll Cardiol* 2:394, 1983.

743. Wiener I. Syndromes of Lown-Ganong-Levine and enhanced atrioventricular nodal conduction. *Am J Cardiol* 52:637, 1983.

744. Abinader EG. Accelerated atrioventricular conduction appearing during acute myocardial infarction. *Chest* 77:632, 1980.

745. Mazuz M, Friedman HS. Significance of prolonged electrocardiographic pauses in sinoatrial disease: Sick sinus syndrome. *Am J Cardiol* 52:485, 1983.

746. Zema MJ, Kligfield P. ECG poor R wave progression. *Arch Intern Med* 142:1145, 1982.

747. DePace NL, Colby J, Hakki A-H, et al. Poor R wave progression in the precordial leads: Clinical implications for the diagnosis of myocardial infarction. *J Am Coll Cardiol* 2:1073, 1983.

748. Zema MJ, Klingfield P. Electrocardiographic tall R waves in the right precordial leads: Vectorcardiographic and electrocardiographic distinction of posterior myocardial infarction from prominent anterior forces in normal subjects. *J Electrocardiol* 17(2):157, 1984.

749. Dell'itallia LJ, Starling MR, O'Rourke RA. Physical examination for exclusion of hemodynamically important right ventricular infarction. *Ann Intern Med* 99:608, 1983.

750. Chou T-C, Fowler NO, Gabel M, et al. Electrocardiographic and hemodynamic changes in experimental right ventricular infarction. *Circulation* 67:1258, 1983.

751. Croft CH, Nicod P, Corbett JR, et al. Detection of acute right ventricular infarction by right precordial electrocardiography. *Am J Cardiol* 50:421, 1982.

752. Zema MJ. The ECG recognition of concomitant left anterior fascicular block and inferior myocardial infarction. *J Electrocardiol* 15(4):401, 1982.

753. Louridas G, Patakas D, Angomachaelis N. Concomitant presence of left anterior hemiblock and inferior myocardial infarction: Electrocardiographic recognition of each entity. *J Electrocardiol* 14(4):365, 1981.

754. Herlitz J, Hjalmarsson A, Waagstein F, et al. The time course in acute myocardial infarction evaluated with precordial mapping and standard ECG. *Clin Cardiol* 6:479, 1983.

755. Engel TR, Caine R, Kowey RR, et al. ST segment elevation with ventricular aneurysm: Results of encircling endocardial ventriculotomy. *J Electrocardiol* 17(1):75, 1984.

756. Jones MR. Atrial myocardial infarction. *Arch Intern Med* 144:573, 1984.

757. Pickering NJ, Engel TR. Atrial coronary angiography. tachyarrhythmias and the Ta segment. *J Electrocardiol* 16(4):325, 1983.

758. Garcin JM, Singer DH. Atrial infarction. *Arch Intern Med* 141:1345, 1981.

759. Farr C, Garver K, Curry RW, et al. Electrocardiographic changes with gastric volvulus. *N Engl J Med* 310:1747, 1984.

760. Ware JA, Magro SA, Luck JC, et al. Conduction system abnormalities in symptomatic mitral valve prolapse: An electrophysiologic analysis of 60 patients. *Am J Cardiol* 53:1075, 1984.

761. Alpert MA, Flaker G. Chronic fascicular block. Recognition, natural history, and therapeutic implications. *Arch Intern Med* 144:799, 1984.

762. Erdberg A, Agmon J. Right axis deviation in acute myocardial infarction: Clinical significance, hospital evolution, and long-term follow-up. *Chest* 85:489, 1984.

763. Reeves WC. ECG criteria for right atrial enlargement. *Arch Intern Med* 143:2155, 1983.
764. Munuswamy K, Alpert MA, Martin RH, et al. Sensitivity and specificity of commonly used electrocardiographic criteria for left atrial enlargement determined by M-mode echocardiography. *Am J Cardiol* 53:829, 1984.
765. Noble LM, Humphrey SB, Monaghan GB. Left ventricular hypertrophy in left bundle branch block. *J Electrocardiol* 17(2):157, 1984.
766. Kishida H, Cole JS, Surawicz B. Negative U wave: A highly specific but poorly understood sign of heart disease. *Am J Cardiol* 49:2030, 1982.
767. Gerson MC, McHenry PL. Resting U wave inversion as a marker of satenosis of the left anterior descending coronary artery. *Am J Med* 69:545, 1980.
768. Kumar S. Persistent ST-segment elevation in hypertrophic subaortic stenosis. *Arch Intern Med* 142:1957, 1982.
769. Karlsson J, Templeton GH, Willerson JT. Relationship between epicardial and S-T segment changes and myocardial metabolism during acute coronary insufficiency. *Circ Res* 32:725, 1973.
770. Prinzmetal M, Ekmekci A, Toyoshima H, et al. Angina pectoris. III. Demonstration of a chemical origin of ST deviation in classic angina pectoris, its variant form, early myocardial infarction, and some non-cardiac conditions. *Am J Cardiol* 3:276, 1959.
771. Prinzmetal M, Toyoshima H, Ekmekci E, et al. Myocardial ischemia. Nature of ischemic electrocardiographic patterns in the mammalian ventricles as determined by intracellular electrographic and metabolic changes. *Am J Cardiol* 8:493, 1961.
772. Feldman T, January CT. ECG changes in pneumothorax. A unique finding and proposed mechanism. *Chest* 86:143, 1984.
773. Mukharji J, Murray S, Lewis SE, et al. Is anterior ST depression with acute transmural inferior infarction due to posterior infarction? A vectorcardiographic and scintigraphic study. *J Am Coll Cardiol* 4:28, 1984.
774. Gerson MC, Phillips JF, Morris SN, et al. Exercise-induced U wave inversion as a marker of stenosis of the left anterior descending coronary artery. *Circulation* 60:1014, 1979.
775. Arvan S, Varat M. Persistent ST-segment elevation and left ventricular wall abnormalities: A 2-dimensional echocardiographic study. *Am J Cardiol* 53:1542, 1984.
776. Bekheit SG, Ali AA, Deglin SM, et al. Analysis of QT interval in patients with mitral valve prolapse. *Chest* 81:620, 1982.

777. Pipberger HV, Chairman. Recommendations for standardization of leads and of specifications for instruments in electrocardiography and vectorcardiography. Report of the committee on electrocardiography, American Heart Association. *Circulation* 52:11, 1975.

778. Geselowitz DB (chairman). Electrical safety standards for electrocardiographic apparatus. Committee Report, American Heart Association. *Circulation* 61:669, 1980.

779. Lepeschkin E. Interrelations between hiccup and the electrocardiogram. *Am J Med* 16:73, 1954.

780. Roberts WC, Silver MA. Norman Jeffries Holter and ambulatory ECG monitoring. *Am J Cardiol* 52:903, 1983.

781. Scheinman MV, Morady F. Invasive cardiac electrophysiologic testing: The current state of the art. *Circulation* 67:1169, 1983.

782. Hammill SC, Pritchett ELC. Simplified esophageal electrocardiography using bipolar recording leads. *Ann Intern Med* 198:14, 1981.

783. Prystowsky EN, Pritchett ELC, Gallagher JJ. Origin of the atrial electrogram recorded from the esophagus. *Circulation* 61:1017, 1980.

784. Giagnoni E, Secchi MB, Wu SC, et al. Prognostic value of exercise EKG testing in asymptomatic normotensive subjects: A prospective matched study. *N Engl J Med* 309:1085, 1983.

785. Quyyumi AA, Wright B, Fox K. Ambulatory electrocardiographic ST segment changes in healthy volunteers. *Br Heart J* 50:460, 1983.

786. Pruitt RD. Symptoms, signs, signals, and shadows. The pathophysiology of angina pectoris—a historical perspective. *Mayo Clin Proc* 58:394, 1983.

787. Strasberg B, Ashley WW, Wyndham CRC, et al. Treadmill exercise testing in the Wolff-Parkinson-White syndrome. *Am J Cardiol* 45:742, 1980.

788. Milliken WA, Pipberger H, Pipberger HV, et al. The impact of an ECG computer analysis program on the cardiologist's interpretation. A cooperative study. *J Electrocardiol* 16(2):141, 1983.

789. Jenkins JM. Automated electrocardiography and arrhythmia monitoring. *Progr Cardiovasc Dis* 25:367, 1983.

790. Rudy Y, Wood R, Plonsey R, et al. The effect of high lung conductivity on electrocardiographic potentials. Results from human subjects undergoing bronchopulmonary lavage. *Circulation* 65:440, 1982.

791. Spodick DH. "Low voltage ECG" and pericardial effusion: Practical and conceptual problems. *Chest* 75:113, 1979.

792. Unverferth DV, Williams TE, Fulkerson PK. Electrocardiographic voltage in pericardial effusion. *Chest* 75:157, 1979.

793. Casale PN, Devereux RB, Kligfield P, et al. Pericardial effusion: Relation of clinical, echocardiographic, and electrocardiographic findings. *J Electrocardiol* 17(2):123, 1984.
794. Parameswaran R, Maniet AR, Goldberg SE, et al. Low electrocardiographic voltage in pericardial effusion. *Chest* 85:631, 1984.
795. Mason JW. Drug therapy: Amiodarone. *N Engl J Med* 316:455, (February 19) 1983.
796. Engler RL, Smith P, LeWinter M, et al. The electrocardiogram in asymmetric septal hypertrophy. *Chest* 75:167, 1979.
797. Gould L, Reddy CVR, Kollali M, et al. Electrocardiographic normalization after cerebral vascular accident. *J Electrocardiol* 14(2):191, 1981.
798. Schwartz PJ. The idiopathic long QT syndrome. *Ann Intern Med* 99:561, 1983.
799. Brodsky M, Wu D, Denes P, et al. Arrhythmias documented by 24 hour continuous electrocardiographic monitoring in 50 male medical students without apparent heart diseae. *Am J Cardiol* 39:390, 1977.
800. Zepelli P, Piarami M, Sessara M, et al. T wave abnormalities in top-ranking athletes: Effects of isoproterenol, atropine, and physical exercise. *Am Heart J* 100:213, 1980.
801. Nishimura T, Kambara H, Chen C-H, et al. Noninvasive assessment of T wave abnormalities on precordial electrocardiograms in middle-aged professional bicyclists. *J Electrocardiol* 14(4):357, 1981.
802. Atterhogand J-H, Malmberg P. Prevalence of primary T-wave changes in young men and their relationship to psychologic and anthropometric data. *Clin Cardiol* 4:91, 1981.
803. Greene HL, Ryan PF, McKusick VA. Profound first degree atrioventricular block. *Chest* 74:212, 1978.
804. Deedwania PC, Swiryn S, Dhingra RC, et al. Nocturnal atrioventricular block as a manifestation of sleep apnea syndrome. *Chest* 76:319, 1979.
805. Gunteroth WG. Sleep apnea and QT interval prolongation—a particularly lethal combination. *Am Heart J* 98:674, 1979.
806. Amaizumi T. Arrhythmias in sleep apnea. *Am Heart J* 100:513, 1980.
807. Drown KF, Prystowsky E, Heger JJ, et al. Prolongation of the QT interval in man during sleep. *Am J Cardiol* 52:55, 1983.
808. Leistner HL, Haddad GG, Lai TL, et al. Heart rate pattern during sleep in an infant with congenital prolongation of the Q-T interval (Romano-Ward syndrome). *Chest* 84:191, 1983.
809. Guilleminault C, Conolly SJ, Winkle RA. Cardiac arrhythmias and conduction disturbances during sleep in 400 patients with sleep apnea syndrome. *Am J Cardiol* 52:490, 1983.

810. Tzivoni D, Stern S. Electrocardiographic pattern during sleep in healthy subjects and in patients with ischemic heart disease. *J Electrocardiol* 6(3):225, 1973.

811. Miller WP. Cardiac arrhythmias and conduction disturbances in the sleep apnea syndrome: Prevalence and significance. *Am J Med* 73:317, 1982.

812. Reuler JB. Hypothermia: pathophysiology, clinical settings, and management. *Ann Intern Med* 89:519, 1978.

813. Emslie-Smith D, Sladden GE, Sterling GR. The significance of changes in the electroardiogram in hypothermia. *Br Heart J* 21:343, 1959.

814. Osborn JJ. Experimental hypothermia: Respiratory and blood pH changes in relation to cardiac function. *Am J Physiol* 175:389, 1953.

815. Gunton RW, Scott JW, Lougheed WM, et al. Changes in cardiac rhythm and in the form of the electrocardiogram resulting from induced hypothermia in man. *Am Heart J* 52:419, 1956.

816. Dodge HT, Grant RP. Mechanisms of QRS prolongation in man. Right ventricular conduction defects. *Am J Med* 21:534, 1956.

817. Bough EW, Boden WF, Korr KS, et al. Left ventricular asynergy in electrocardiographic "posterior" myocardial infarction. *J Am Coll Cardiol* 4:209, 1984.

818. Surawicz B, Knoebel SB. Long QT: Good, bad, or indifferent. *J Am Coll Cardiol* 4:398, 1984.

819. Lown B, Ganong WF, Levine SA. The syndrome of short P-R interval, normal QRS complex, and paroxysmal rapid heart action. *Circulation* 5:693, 1952.

820. Sridharan MR, Flowers NC. Computerized electrocardiographic analysis. *Mod Conc Cardiovasc Dis* 53:37, 1984.

821. Spirito P, Maron BJ, Bonow RO, et al. The prevalence and significance of abnormal S-T segment response to exercise in a young athletic population. *Am J Cardiol* 51:1663, 1983.

822. Kunkes SH, Pichard AD, Smith H Jr, et al. Silent ST segment deviations and extent of coronary artery disease. *Am Heart J* 100:813, 1980.

823. Armstrong WF, Jordan JW, Morris SN, et al. Prevalence and magnitude of S-T segment and T wave abnormalities in normal men during continuous ambulatory electrocardiography. *Am J Cardiol* 49:1638, 1982.

824. Balady GJ, Cadigan JB, Ryan TJ. Electrocardiogram of the athlete: An analysis of 289 professional football players. *Am J Cardiol* 53:1339, 1984.

825. Cheng TC. Electrical alternans. An association with coronary spasm. *Arch Intern Med* 143:1052, 1983.

826. Wayne VS, Bishop RL, Spodick DH. Exercise-induced ST-segment alternans. *Chest* 83:824, 1983.
827. Wenger NK. The ECG in normal pregnancy. *Arch Intern Med* 142:1088, 1982.
828. Ziegler RF. *Electrocardiographic Studies in Normal Infants and Children.* Springfield: Charles C. Thomas, 1951.
829. Zack PM, Wiens RD, Kennedy HL. Left-axis deviation and obesity: The United States Health and Nutrition Examination Survey. *Am J Cardiol* 53:1129, 1984.
830. Dickinson BF, Scott O. Ambulatory electrocardiographic monitoring in 100 healthy teenage boys. *Br Heart J* 51:179, 1984.
831. Grant RP, Dodge HT. Mechanisms of QRS prolongation in man. Left ventricular conduction disturbances. *Am J Med* 20:834, 1956.
832. McNulty JH, Rahimtoola S. Bundle branch block. *Progr Cardiovasc Dis* 26:333, 1984.
833. Pruitt RD, Essex HE, Burchell HB. Studies on the spread of excitation through the ventricular myocardium. *Circulation* 3:418, 1951.
834. Gressard A. Left bundle branch block with left axis deviation: An electrophysiologic approach. *Am J Cardiol* 52:1013, 1983.
835. Deanfield JE, Selwyn AP, Chierchia S, et al. Myocardial ischaemia during daily life in patients with stable angina: Its relation to symptoms and heart rate changes. *Lancet* 2:753, 1983.
836. Miller WP. Cardiac arrhythmias and conduction disturbances in the sleep apnea syndrome: Prevalence and significance. *Am J Med* 73:317, 1984.
837. Cohn PF. When is concern about silent myocardial ischemia justified? *Ann Intern Med* 100:597, 1984.
838. Leighton RF, Fraker TD. Silent myocardial ischemia: Concern is justified for the patient with known coronary artery disease. *Ann Intern Med* 100:599, 1984.
839. Little WC, Rogers EW, Sodums MT. Mechanism of anterior ST segment depression during acute inferior myocardial infarction: Observations during coronary thrombolysis. *Ann Intern Med* 100:226, 1984.
840. Perlman LV, Ostrander LD Jr, Keller JB, et al. An epidemiologic study of first degree atrioventricular block in Tecumseh, Michigan. *Chest* 23:40, 1971.
841. Rodstein M, Brown M, Wolloch L. First degree atrioventricular heart block in the aged. *Geriatrics* 23:159, 1968.
842. Heller GV, Aroesty J, McKay RG, et al. The pacing stress test: A reexamination of the relation between coronary artery disease and pacing-electrocardiographic changes. *Am J Cardiol* 54:50, 1984.

843. Lindsay J Jr, Dewey RC, Talesnick BS, et al. Relation of ST-segment elevation after healing of myocardial infarction to the presence of left ventricular aneurysm. *Am J Cardiol* 54:84, 1984.

844. Sarma JSM, Sarma RJ, Bilitch M, et al. An exponential formula for heart rate dependence of QT interval during exercise and cardiac pacing in humans: Reevaluation of Bazett's formula. *Am J Cardiol* 54:103, 1984.

845. Rao PS, Thapar MK, Harp RJ. Racial variations in electrocardiograms and vectorcardiograms between black and white children and their genesis. *J Electrocardiol* 17(3):239, 1984.

846. Wenger NK, Hurst JW, Strozier VN. Electrocardiographic changes in pregnancy. *Am J Cardiol* 13:774, 1964.

847. Bachman S, Sparrow D, Smith LK. Effect of aging on the electrocardiogram. *Am J Cardiol* 48:513, 1981.

848. Fisch C. Electrocardiogram in the aged: An independent marker of heart disease? *Am J Med* 70:4, 1981.

849. Schwartz DB, Schamroth L. Effects of pregnancy on the frontal plane QRS axis. *J Electrocardiol* 12(3):279, 1979.

850. Caruth JE, Mirvis SB, Brogan DR, et al. The electrocardiogram in normal pregnancy. *Am Heart J* 102:1075, 1981.

851. Barolsky SN, Gilbert CA, Faruqui A, et al. Differences in electrocardiographic response to exercise of men and women: A non-Bayesian factor. *Circulation* 60:1021, 1979.

852. Sketch MH, Mohiuddin SM, Lynch JD, et al. Significant sex differences in the correlation of electrocardiographic exercise testing and coronary arteriograms. *Am J Cardiol* 36:169, 1975.

853. Plonsey R. A contemporary view of the ventricular gradient of Wilson. *J Electrocardiol* 12(4):337, 1979.

854. Schaefer H. The general order of excitation and recovery. *Ann NY Acad Sci* 65:743, 1957.

855. Gardberg M, Rosen IL. The ventricular gradient of Wilson. *Ann NY Acad Sci* 65:873, 1957.

856. Scher AM, Young AC. Ventricular depolarization and the genesis of QRS. *Ann NY Acad Sci* 65:768, 1957.

857. Haraphongse M, Tanomsup S, Jugdutt BI. Inferior ST segment depression during acute anterior myocardial infarction: Clinical and angiographic correlations. *J Am Coll Cardiol* 4:467, 1984.

858. Forman MB, Goodin J, Phelan B, et al. Electrocardiographic changes associated with isolated right ventricular infarction. *J Am Coll Cardiol* 4:640, 1984.

859. Sridharan MR, Horan LG. Electrocardiographic J Wave of hypercal-cemia. *Am J Cardiol* 54:672, 1984.
860. Wenckebach KF. Beitragezur Kenntnis der menschlichen Herztatigkeit. *Arch fur Anatomie und Physiol (Phys. Abteil.)* 297, 1906.
861. Murphy ML, Thenabadu N, Blue LR, et al. Descriptive characteristics of the electrocardiogram from autopsied men free of cardiopulmonary disease—a basis for evaluating criteria for ventricular hypertrophy. *Am J Cardiol* 52:1361, 1983.
862. Mazzoleni A, Hagan AD, Glover MU, et al. On the relationship between Q waves in leads II and aVF and inferior-posterior wall motion abnormalities. *J Electrocardiol* 16(4):367, 1983.
863. Murphy ML, Thenabadu PN, de Soyza N, et al. Reevaluation of electrocardiographic criteria for left, right, and combined cardiac ventricular hypertrophy. *Am J Cardiol* 53:1140, 1984.
864. Mautner RK, Siegel LA, Giles TD, et al. Electrocardiographic changes in acute pancreatitis. *Southern Med J* 75:317, 1982.
865. Gardin JM, Belic N, Singer DH. Pseudoarrhythmias in ambulatory ECG monitoring. *Arch Intern Med* 139:809, 1979.
866. Kumar SP, Yans J, Kwatra M. Unusual artifacts in electrocardiographic monitoring. *J Electrocardiol* 12(3):295, 1979.
867. Agarwal SK. An unusual ECG artifact—results of a faulty recorder. *J Am Med Assoc* 242:617, 1979.
868. James WC. Electrocardiographic artifacts caused by defective marker circuitry. *J Am Med Assoc* 247:1564, 1982.
869. Groeger JS, Miodownik S, Howland WS. ECG infusion artifact. *Chest* 85:143, 1984.
870. Pilcher GF, Cook AJ, Johnston BL, et al. Twenty-four hour continuous electrocardiography during exercise and free activity in 80 apparently healthy runners. *Am J Cardiol* 52:859, 1983.
871. Fuchs RM, Achuff SC, Grunwald L, et al. Electrocardiographic localization of coronary narrowings: Studies during myocardial ischemia and infarction in patients with one-vessel disease. *Circulation* 66:1168, 1982.
872. Movahed A, Becker LC. Electrocardiographic changes of acute lateral wall myocardial infarction: A reappraisal based on scintigraphic localization of the infarct (The heart's beat, J Physiol 8:229, 1887). *J Am Coll Cardiol* 4:660, 1984.
873. Laslett LJ, Amsterdam EA. Management of the asymptomatic subject with an abnormal exercise ECG. *J Am Med Assoc* 252:1744, 1984.

874. Tendera M, Campbell WB. Significance of early and late anterior precordial ST segment depression in inferior myocardial infarction. *Am J Cardiol* 54:994, 1984.

875. Crawford MH, O'Rourke R, Grover FL. Mechanism of inferior electrocardiographic ST segment depression during anterior myocardial infarction in a baboon model. *Am J Cardiol* 54:1114, 1984.

876. Kawataki M, Kashima R, Toda W, et al. Relation between QT interval and heart rate. Applications and limitation of Bazett's formula. *J Electrocardiol* 17(4):371, 1984.

877. Deanfield JE, Shea M, Ribiero P, et al. Transient ST-segment depression as a marker of myocardial ischemia during daily life. *Am J Cardiol* 54:1195, 1985.

878. Edwards BS, Edwards WD, Edwards JE. Ventricular septal rupture complicating acute myocardial infarction: Identification of simple and complex types of 53 autopsied hearts. *Am J Cardiol* 54:1201, 1984.

879. Boden WE, Bough EW, Korr KS, et al. Inferoseptal myocardial infarction: Another cause of precordial ST-segment depression in transmural inferior wall myocardial infarction. *Am J Cardiol* 54:1216, 1984.

880. Packer DL, Coltorti F, Smith MS, et al. Sudden death after left stellectomy in the long QT syndrome. *Am J Cardiol* 54:1365, 1984.

881. Alpert JS. Association between arrhythmias and mitral valve prolapse. *Arch Intern Med* 144:2333, 1984.

882. Kramer HM, Kligfield P, Devereaux RB, et al. Arrhythmias in mitral valve prolapse. *Arch Intern Med* 144:2360, 1984.

883. Chava NR. ECG in diabetic ketoacidosis. *Arch Intern Med* 144:2379, 1984.

884. Moss AJ, Schwartz PJ, Crampton RS, et al. The long QT syndrome: A prospective international study. *Circulation* 71:1721, 1985.

885. Ludmer PL, Goldschlager N. Cardiac pacing in the 1980s. *N Engl J Med* 311:1671, 1985.

886. Kafka H, Burggraf GW, Milliken JA. Electrocardiographic diagnosis of left ventricular hypertrophy in the presence of left bundle branch block: An echocardiographic study. *Am J Cardiol* 55:103, 1985.

887. Bedell SE, Aronson MD. Late development of electrocardiographic abnormalities after a stroke. *Southern Med J* 78:218, 1985.

888. Biel SI, Kleiger RE. Ventricular premature complexes in the early diagnosis of acute myocardial infarction. *Southern Med J* 78:710, 1985.

889. Guilleminault C, Pool P, Motta J, et al. Sinus arrest during REM sleep in young adults. *N Engl J Med* 311:1006, 1984.

890. Green LS, Lux RL, Haws CW, et al. Effects of age, sex, and body habitus on QRS and ST-T potential maps of 1100 normal subjects. *Circulation* 71:244, 1985.

891. Meijler FL. Atrioventricular conduction versus heart size from mouse to whale. *J Am Coll Cardiol* 5:363, 1985.

892. deLuna AB, de Ribot RF, Trilla E, et al. Electrocardiographic and vectorcardiographic study of interatrial conduction disturbances with left atrial retrograde conduction. *J Electrocardiol* 18(1):1–14, 1985.

893. Gulamhusein S, Yee R, Ko PT, et al. Electrocardiographic criteria for differentiating aberrancy and ventriulcar extrasystole in chronic atrial fibrillation: Validation by intracardiac recordings. *J Electrocardiol* 18(1):41, 1985.

894. Kulbertus H, Rigo P, Legrand V. Right ventricular infarction: Pathophysiology, diagnosis, clinical course, and treatment. *Mod Conc Cardiovasc Dis* 54:15, 1985.

895. Scherlag BJ, Gunn CS, Berbari EJ, et al. Peri-infarction block (1950)—late potentials (1980): Their relationship, significance, and diagnostic implications. *Am J Cardiol* 55:839, 1985.

896. Klein HO, Beker B, Sarelim , et al. Unusual QRS morphology associated with transvenous pacemakers. The pseudo RBBB pattern. *Chest* 87:517, 1985.

897. Rajala SA, Geiger UKM, Haavisto MV, et al. Electrocardiogram, clinical findings, and chest x-ray in persons aged 85 years or older. *Am J Cardiol* 55:1175, 1985.

898. Oreto G, Buzza F, Klein HO, et al. Asynchronous intraventricular recovery as a basis for "supernormality." *J Electrocardiol* 18(2):195, 1985.

899. Fulton DR, Chung KJ, Tabakin BS, et al. Ventricular tachycardia in children without heart disease. *Am J Cardiol* 55:1328, 1985.

900. Selzer A, Rokeach S. Clinical, electrocardiographic, and ventriculographic consequences of isolated occlusion of the right coronary artery. *Am J Med* 78:749, 1985.

901. Moorman JR. Digitalis toxicity at Duke Hospital. *Southern Med J* 78:561, 1985.

902. Rotman M, Triebwasser JH. A clinical and follow-up study of right and left bundle branch block. *Circulation* 51:477, 1975.

903. Dec GW Jr, Stern TA, Welch C. The effects of electroconvulsive therapy on serial electrocardiograms and serum cardiac enzyme values. A prospective study of depressed hospitalized inpatients. *J Am Med Assoc* 253:2525, 1985.

904. Zema MJ. Q wave, ST segment, and T wave myocardial infarction. Useful clinical distinction. *Am J Med* 78:391, 1985.

905. Brush JE Jr, Brand DA, Acampora D, et al. Use of the initial electrocardiogram to predict in-hospital complications of acute myocardial infarction. *N Engl J Med* 312:1137, 1985.

906. Willems JL (moderator). Criteria for intraventricular conduction disturbances and pre-excitation. World Health Organization/International Society and Federation for Cardiology Task Force Ad Hoc. *J Am Coll Cardiol* 5:1261, 1985.

907. Fisch C (moderator). Clinical electrophysiology and electrocardiography. *J Am Coll Cardiol* 6:6B, 1985.

908. Surawicz B. Basic principles of electrophysiology. *J Am Coll Cardiol* 6:28B, 1985.

909. Mirvis DM, Ingram L, Holly MK, et al. Electrocardiographic effects of experimental nontransmural myocardial infarction. *Circulation* 71:1206, 1985.

910. Turi ZG, et al. Electrocardiographic, enzymatic and scintigraphic criteria of acute myocardial infarction as determined from a study of 726 patients (a MILIS study). Multicenter investigation of the limitation of infarct size. *Am J Cardiol* 55:1463, 1985.

911. Moorman JR, Pritchett ELC. The arrhythmias of digitalis intoxication. *Arch Intern Med* 145:1289, 1985.

912. Huston TP, Puffer JC, Rodney WM. The athletic heart syndrome. *N Engl J Med* 313:2432, 1985.

913. Bean WB. Origin of the term "internal medicine." *N Engl J Med* 306:182, 1982.

914. Minsky M. *The Society of the Mind. New York*: Simon and Schuster, 1986.

915. Allessie MA, Lammers WJEP, Bonke IM, et al. Intra-atrial reentry as a mechanism for atrial flutter induced by acetylcholine and rapid pacing in the dog. *Circulation* 70:123, 1984.

916. Roland CG. *William Osler's The Master Word In Medicine*. Springfield, Illinois: Charles C. Thomas, 1972.

917. Mackenzie J. *Diseases of the Heart*, 4th ed. London: Oxford Medical Publ., 1925.

918. Boineau JP. Atrial flutter, a synthesis of concepts. *Circulation* 72:249, 1985.

919. Grant RP. The relationship of unipolar chest leads to the electrical field of the heart. *Circulation* 1:878, 1950.

920. Rosenthal J, Rosenthal M. True colors. What's licorice and bisque and jalapeno all over? *The Atlantic Monthly* 266:18, 1990.

921. Mandel WJ. *Cardiac Arrhythmias. Their Mechanisms, Diagnosis and Management*, 2nd ed. Philadelphia: J. B. Lippincott, 1987.

922. Lown B, Marcus F, Levine HD. Digitalis and atrial tachycardia with block. *N Engl J Med* 260:301, 1959.

923. Krikler DM. The search for Samojloff: A Russian physiologist in times of change. *Br Med J* 295:1624, 1987.

924. Herrick JB. Clinical features of sudden obstruction of the coronary arteries. *J Am Med Assoc* 59:2015, 1912.

925. Grant RP. Spatial vector electrocardiography. A method for calculating the spatial electrical vectors of the heart from conventional leads. *Circulation* 2:676, 1950.

926. Wilson FN, Macleod AG, Barker PS, et al. The electrocardiogram in myocardial infarction with particular reference to the initial deflections in the ventricular complex. *Heart* 16:155, 1933.

927. Sodi-Pallares D, Medrano G, De Micheli A, et al. Unipolar QS morphology and Purkinje potential of the free left ventricular wall. The concept of the electrical endocardium. *Circulation* 23:836, 1963.

928. Sodi-Pallares D, Calder RM. *New Bases of Electrocardiography*. St. Louis: C. V. Mosby, 1956.

929. Frantz MR. Method and theory of monophasic action potential recording. *Progr Cardiovasc Dis* 33:347, 1991.

930. Einthoven W, Fahr G, de Waart A. On the direction and manifest size of the variations of potential in the human heart and on the influence of the position of the heart on the form of the electrocardiogram. Pfluger's Arch. f. d. ges. Physiol. 150:275-315, 1913. Translated by Hebel E. Hoff and Paul Seklj. *Am Heart J* 40:163, 1950.

931. Dimond EG, Berry F. Transmission of electrocardiographic signals over telephone circuits. *Am Heart J* 46:906, 1953.

932. Chung K-Y, Walsh TJ, Massie E. Wolff-Parkinson-White syndrome. *Am Heart J* 69:116, 1965.

933. Wu D, Denes P, Dingra RC, et al. Electrophysiologic and clinical observations in patients. *Circulation* 53:456, 1976.

934. Ashman R, Hull E. *Essentials of Electrocardiography*, 2nd ed. New York: The Macmillan Company, 1941.

935. Lepeschkin E. *Modern Electrocardiography*. Baltimore: Williams and Wilkins, 1951.

936. Lazzara R. Cellular basis for the U wave and its translation to the surface ECG. *J Electrocardiol* Supplement:44, 1991.

937. Willems, et al. The diagnostic performance of computer programs for the interpretation of electrocardiograms. *N Engl J Med* 325:1767, 1991.

938. Alpert MA, Munuswamy K. Electrocardiographic diagnosis of left atrial enlargement. *Arch Intern Med* 149:1161, 1989.

939. Sokolow MA, Friedlander RD. The normal unipolar precordial and limb lead electrocardiogram. *Am Heart J* 38:665, 1956.

940. Habbab MA, El-Sherif N. Drug-induced torsades de pointes: Role of early after-depolarizations and dispersion of repolarization. *Am J Med* 89:241, 1990.

941. Sasyniuk BI, Valois M, Toy W. Recent advances in understanding the mechanisms of drug-induced torsades des pointes arrhythmias. *Am J Cardiol* 64:29J, 1989.

942. Cowan JC, Yusoff K, Moore M, et al. Importance of lead selection in QT interval measurement. *Am J Cardiol* 61:83, 1988.

943. Wallis DE, Littman WJ, Scanlon PJ, et al. The effect of elevated intra-cranial pressure on the canine electrocardiogram. *J Electrocardiol* 20(2):154, 1987.

944. Nakamura Y, Kaseno K, Kubo T. Transient ST segment elevation in subarachnoid hemorrhage. *J Electrocardiol* 22(2):133, 1989.

945. Koskelo P, Pursar S, Sipila W. Subendocardial hemorrhage and E.C.G. changes in intracranial bleeding. *Br Med J* 1:1479, 1964.

946. Sanchez-Cascos A, Deuchar D. The P wave in atrial septal defect. *Br Heart J* 25:202, 1963.

947. Cabrera E, Monroy J. Systolic and diastolic loading of the heart. II. Electrocardiographic data. *Am Heart J* 43:661, 1952.

948. Hersch C. Electrocardiographic changes in subarachnoid hemorrhage, meningitis, and intracranial space-occupying lesions. *Br Heart J* 26:785, 1964.

949. McKenna WJ, Borggrefe M, England D, et al. The natural history of left ventricular hypertrophy in hypertrophic cardiomyopathy: An electrocardiographic study. *Circulation* 66:1233, 1966.

950. Jackman WM, Wang XZ, et al. Catheter ablation of accessory atrioventricular pathways (Wolff-Parkinson-White syndrome) by radiofrequency current. *N Engl J Med* 324:1612, 1991.

951. Lange RA, Cigarroa RG, et al. Cocaine induced coronary artery vaso-constriction. *N Engl J Med* 321:1557, 1989.

952. Sherief HT, Carpientier RG. Electrophysiologic mechanisms of cocaine-induced cardiac arrest. *J Electrocardiol* 24(3):247, 1991.
953. Lewis W. AIDS: cardiac findings from 115 autopsies. *Progr Cardiovasc Dis* 32:207, 1989.
954. Nelson SD, Kou WH, et al. Significance of ST depression during paroxysmal supraventricular tachycardia. *Am J Cardiol* 12:383, 1988.
955. Bayes de Luna A, Carrio I, Subirana MT, et al. Electrophysiological mechanisms of the S1,S2,S3 electrocardiographic morphology. *J Electrocardiol* 20(1):38, 1987.
956. Hurst JW. *Ventricular Electrocardiography*. Lippincott, Philadelphia, 1991; Gover, New York London.
957. Burnum JF. Medical diagnosis through semiotics: giving meaning to the sign. *Ann Int Med* 119:939, 1993.

Index